Facial Diagnosis For Everyone

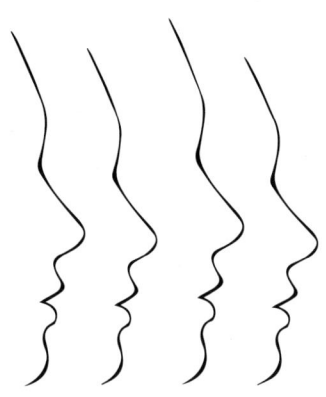

Facial Diagnosis For Everyone

Practical Solutions Using Herbs, Cell Salts, and Homeopathy

DAVID R. CARD

Kalindi Press
Chino Valley, Arizona

© 2025, David R. Card

All rights reserved. No part of this book may be reproduced in any manner without written permission from the publisher, except in the case of quotes used in critical articles and reviews.

Cover design: Hohm Press
Layout and design: Becky Fulker, Kubera Book Design

print book ISBN: 978-1-935826-62-0

eBook ISBN: 978-1-935826-63-7

Library of Congress Control Number: 2025930398

Kalindi Press
PO Box 4410
Chino Valley, AZ 86323
800-381-2700
www.kalindipress.com

This book was printed in China on recycled paper using soy ink.

Disclaimer: The material in this book is intended for educational purposes only, and as such is not meant to be a substitute for professional medical intervention or used to treat or diagnose diseases. In any use of cell salts or other approaches discussed in this book, please apply common sense and consult a qualified, licensed health care professional.

Table of Contents

	Introduction To Facial Diagnosis	vii
	Chinese Perspective on the Face	viii
	Personal Care Tools	ix
	Faces and their Meanings	x
Faces:	Depression and Anxiety	1
	Spine	7
	Thyroid (Hyperthyroid, Hypothyroid, and Goiter)	12
	Heart	22
	Lungs (Asthma, Bronchitis, Pneumonia)	27
	Kidneys	34
	Adrenals: Stress	40
	Stomach (Stomach and Stomach Ulcers)	45
	Liver	51
	Gallbladder	57
	Pancreas (Blood Sugar and Type II Diabetes)	61
	Colon: Large Intestine	69
	Aging	77
	Men's Health: Prostate	81
	Women's Health: Child-bearing through Menopause	87

Special Thanks to artists Monique Ordonez and Emily Decker

Introduction to Facial Diagnosis

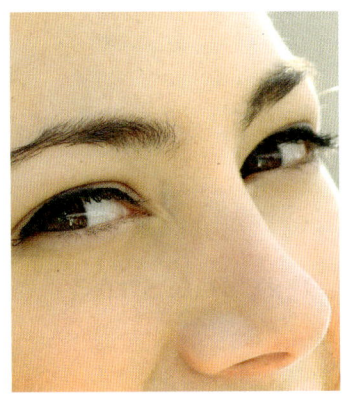

Facial diagnosis is the art of looking at a person's face to discover what organ system is not functioning properly, or what disease process may be at work. Our face reflects the health of our body, and when unwanted blemishes, lines, colors, etc. are present, these may be signs of disfunction.

The health of the body is dependent upon our organs, which reflects in our face. All things are connected inside and out; each part of our body (organs, tissues) is connected with our emotional state as well. So, emotions are also revealed in the face. It's like anything else, we just have look closer to see what's there.

As a society we tend to be over-concerned with appearance. Using modern technology, doctors can remove superficial blemishes through laser treatments, creams, injections, and even surgeries. Often, people are dissatisfied with these treatments, as the problem tends to resurface in the same spot.

It's important to remove the cause of the facial signs, naturally, through good nutrition and using natural supplements for support. Improving overall health and well-being reduces the cause of our facial signs—the internal disfunctions—and will negate the need for facial surgeries or treatments, except in the case of injuries. While diet is important, the natural supplements included in this book are quite effective in supporting organ function as well as mental/emotional health. They include **herbs, homeopathic medicines, and cell salts (for mineral deficiency).** The cell salt explanations will add a different perspective on physical, emotional, or mental symptoms as well. **Using these and other personal care tools will help balance and support organ function for better overall health.**

The next page shows the Chinese diagnosing perspective of the face. It is a tool they have used for thousands of years. Their concept of the associated organs is somewhat different than the western point of view. However, they **do not rely upon facial diagnosis alone for the final assessment of a disease.** There are other body diagnostic tools available from several other cultures and masters' experiences. Some of the facial, or body signs, may or may not equate to a medical diagnosis.

The Facial Diagnosis Book facial renderings are the extremes and don't represent a normal face. An average face may present several layers of organ weakness. **This perspective of the face provides hints that must be taken with other signs and symptoms** to determine the course to follow. Use this book to help assess a person's health in reading signs in the face. Remember, one sign is not enough to establish a pattern. It takes several signs and sometimes a medical diagnosis. One can help themselves by natural means, but **must rely upon a healthcare professional for diagnosis.** Only doctors can legally diagnose or treat conditions or disease.

Important:
- This book is not designed to diagnose or treat any condition or disease; it only represents an historical perspective.
- Always consult a doctor if there is a suspected condition or disease.
- The selection of herbs, homeopathic, cell salts, diet, and nutrition can be used alongside your over-the-counter or prescription medicines.
- Consult a doctor for use in pregnancy or while nursing.

Facial Diagnosis Using the Chinese Perspective of the Face

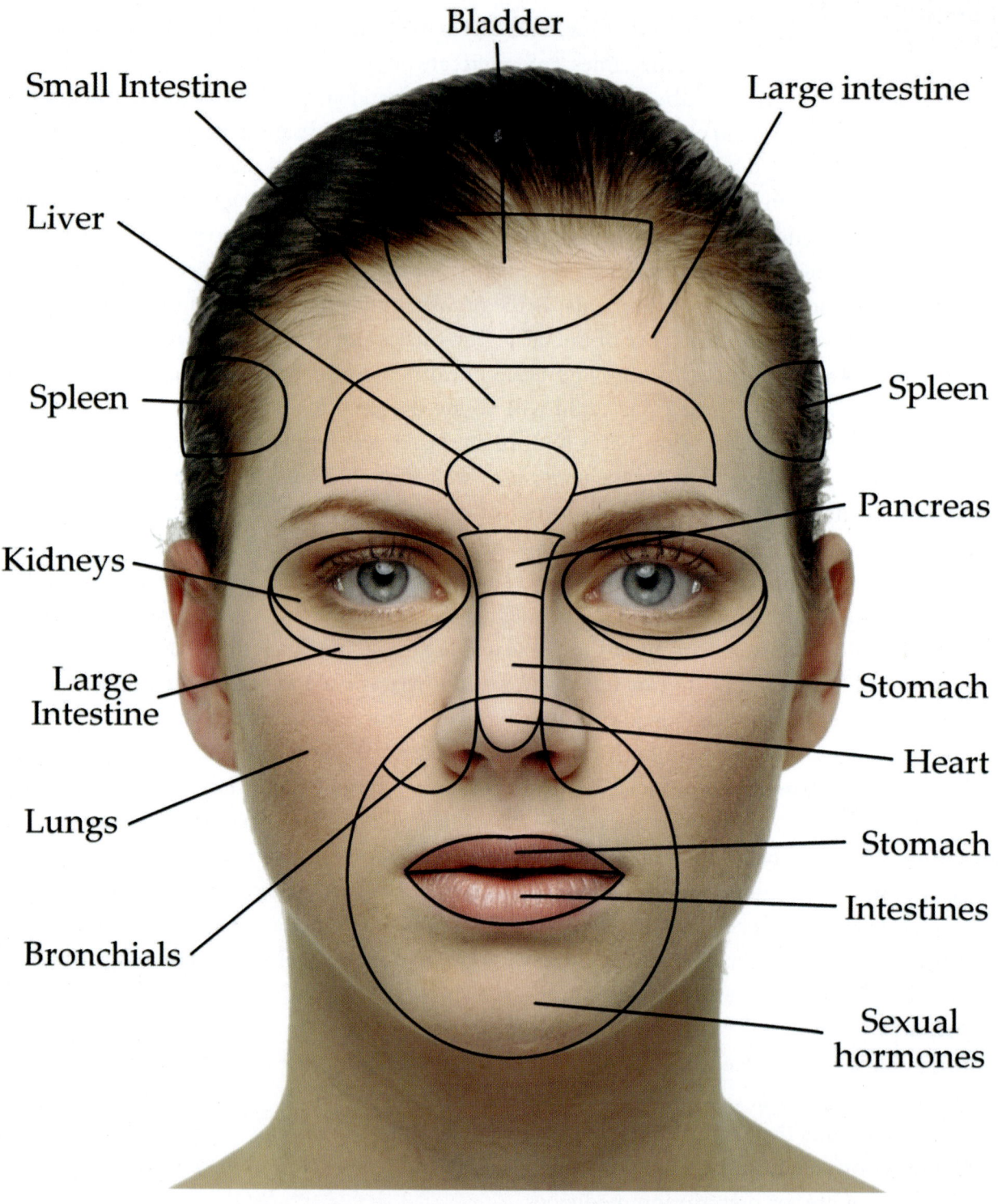

viii FACIAL DIAGNOSIS USING THE CHINESE PERSPECTIVE OF THE FACE

Personal Care Tools

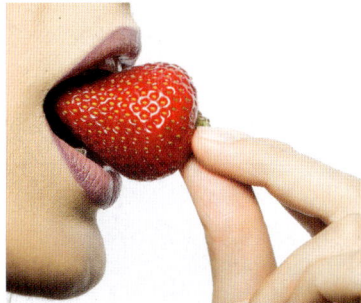

Diet – Nourishment
Diet is important to maintain excellent health. Without it you can't get healthy.

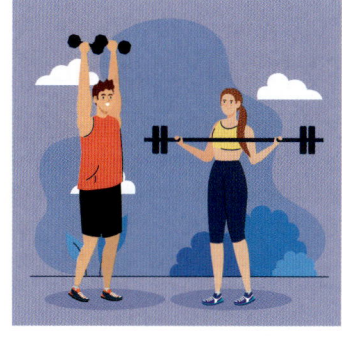

Exercise
Exercise helps us to move the lymphatic system (immune health) to help get rid of metabolic wastes.

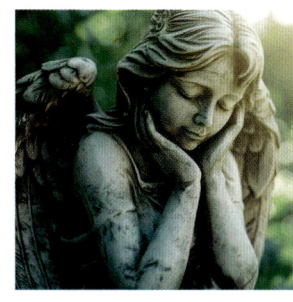

Spiritual Emotional
We are connected to each other and to God. Our emotions and spirit affect our health.

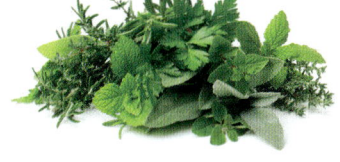

Herbs
Herbs are foods that contain nutrients to bring us into balance.

Homeopathy
Homeopathy is a very large healthcare system worldwide and provides tools to help us regain health and balance.

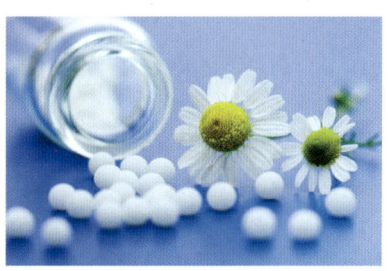

Cell Salts
Cell salts are minerals that help create balance by providing the cells the right minerals to get healthy.

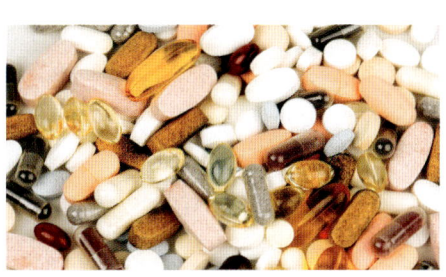

Nutritional Supplements
Supplements can help us overcome nutritional deficiencies caused by stress, medications, pollution, and other causes.

Faces and their Meanings in our Lives

All that we experience is here for our learning and growth. The following expressions are the focus of each face we will be talking about:

- **Depression** is the opportunity to examine our life and change our direction.

- The **Spine** represents your support for your emotional and physical body.

- The **Thyroid** signifies how you metabolize live, understanding your experiences.

- The **Heart** helps you stay in balance between your spiritual and physical existence.

- **Lungs** represent our contact to the physical world.

- **Kidneys** facilitate controlling our fear and releasing toxins.

- **Adrenals** are the key to managing stress and represent our zest for life.

- The **Stomach** represents our absorbing life and finding joy, including food.

- The **Liver** represents communicating in a healthy manner to avoid anger that may turn into depression.

- The **Gallbladder** embodies our courage to get beyond the bitterness of life's experiences.

- **Pancreas** represents the balance between our metabolism (endocrine) and digestion (exocrine).

- The **Colon** symbolizes our need to release the unneeded things in life.

- **Aging** happens – we don't get out of this life alive, but we can be healthy 'til we exit.

- The **Prostate** represents overcoming selfishness and managing our maleness.

- **Women's Hormones** are a symbol of how one finds joy in their femininity.

Depression and Anxiety

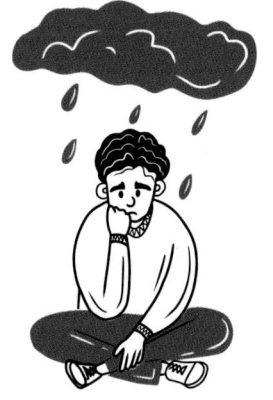

Depression is an important part of life that everyone experiences at one point or another. The causes are many, but as I see it, depression is nature's way of looking at problems and trying to correct them.

Depression means that the balance of life is disturbed, and lets us know that it needs to be fixed. We need to examine our life and fix those areas. **It gives us the opportunity to make positive changes.**

Modern medicine calls depression a brain chemical imbalance of the neurotransmitters. The stigma is that a person is broken, mentally ill, and must be medicated for the rest of their life. Antidepressant medications have major side effects, from emotional numbness to loss of sexual interest. Anti-depressants can be useful for a short time, but create dependence and other various side effects. *The reality is that they actually hinder the healing process.*

Depression disappears when the cause is found and the problem addressed.

The main cause of depression in WOMEN is hormonal imbalances caused by birth control devices, dairy, meat, or other nutritional deficiencies. Premenopausal women may use Vitex or Blessed Thistle herbs. Post-menopausal women can use Eleutherococcus (Siberian Ginseng) and may add Suma. This will help the adrenal glands to produce the proper hormones to function healthily.

Other causes of depression include disturbed digestion, often caused by stress or other factors. The stomach contains more serotonin than the brain! Hence, the term "gut reaction." Use natural digestive enhancers and avoid all stomach acid reducers and neutralizers. **Parasites** can also be a cause with symptoms that include dark circles under the eyes, digestive disturbances, and nervous irritability. This is often seen in children as well.

Heavy metal toxicity. There are several good commercial detoxification products.

Thyroid dysfunction can be a physical cause. Symptoms can include weight gain and lethargy. Use kelp and other natural products to promote healthy thyroid function. Consult a doctor to test the thyroid if this is suspected.

Emotional issues can also lead to depression, due to different emotional traumas specific to the individual. Therefore, it is necessary to use the specific homeopathic remedy in combination with cell salts and supportive herbs or formulas. Symptoms of depression or nervousness may include:

- Anxiety
- Loss of normal pleasures
- Sleep disturbances
- Feeling guilty or worthless
- Exhaustion
- Inability to concentrate
- Loss of appetite
- Suicidal thoughts

Depression and Anxiety Facial Diagnosis

Hair graying early from emotional shock

Ears, strongly flattened upper ear border

Downtrodden appearance to face

Gray skin tones

Sunken cheeks and temples

Eyebrow, one side higher than the other

Eyebrows, wrinkle in an omega shape between the eyebrows

Eyebrows in younger people turn gray early

Eyes dull, restless or nervous

Eyes, slight bluish orbits of eyes

Eyes, sunken with brownish-black circles

Hanging lower eyelids

Root of nose is deeply indented, and if root is small: nervousness

Cheeks, isolated white or pale spots indicate nerve exhaustion

Cheeks, spotty beard growth

Chin pointed and turned downward

Upper lip, small w/corners of the mouth turned downward

Talks in monotones and has a stoic face

Teeth, grinding of

Tongue shakes, and if swollen – nerve inflammation

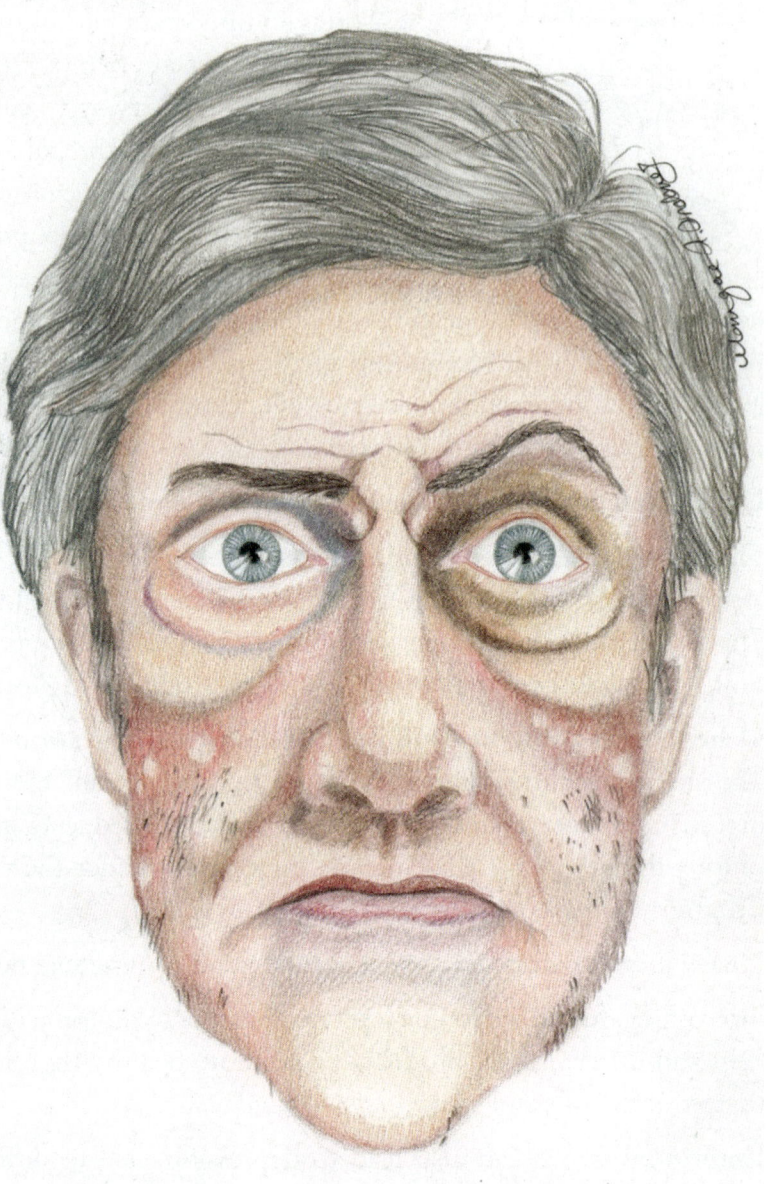

Other Body Depression Signs

Shoulder, one higher than the other

Restlessness can indicate nerve weakness

Walking, unsure, especially on stairs

Writing, cramped, can indicate nervous disturbance

Depression and Anxiety Herbs

These herbs are mostly adaptogenic, herbs that balance stress and energy needs. Other herbs are nervines that support the nervous system.

#1 ZEMBRIN is an extract of sceletium tortosum, called "Kanna," which seems to work to reduce anxiety and depression symptoms well. You should notice positive effects in two to four hours, in my experience. No significant side effects have been reported in thousands of my clients.

American Ginseng is calming, and rejuvenative. Depression from fibromyalgia or chronic fatigue.

Ashwagandha is an adaptogen for those depressed; depression from fibromyalgia.

Black Cohosh is for menopausal depression. Doom and gloom attitude, feeling as if there's a "black cloud" over the head. Can be combined with Vitex.

Damiana is for depression where the sex drive is lowered, especially if related to past sexual abuse.

Eleutherococcus (Siberian Ginseng) is for long-term use in mild depression, exhaustion—e.g., a young executive who drinks recreationally and has trouble sleeping.

Gingko Biloba for mild depression, and depression associated with the elderly, who might also suffer from impaired vision, memory loss, and cognitive problems.

Lavender for depression that is related to PTSD, in which there is a stagnant fixation on a past event and where symptoms can include insomnia, gas, nausea, indigestion.

Lemon Balm is a mild mood elevator. Can help with depression-related insomnia and compromised cognition. Also useful for seasonal affective disorder and mild hypertension.

Albizia is for depression from a broken heart, when the person is consumed with grief. Often combined with Hawthorn flowers and fragrant Rose petals.

Red or White Panax Ginseng is for depression from extreme fatigue, even when too tired to sleep.

Rhodiola is for nervous depression and immune weakness. Can provide energy without overstimulation. Also improves circulation, especially to the head.

Schizandra can help with depression related to coffee-deprivation. Also for depression related to liver issues. Strengthens the hypothalamus, pituitary, and adrenals. Energizes the entire nervous

St. John's Wort is for mild to medium depression, lack of day-to-day joy. Also for seasonal-affective disorder (with lemon balm).

Depression and Anxiety Homeopathic Medicines

From Dr. Robin Murphy Materia Medica

30c potencies taken once a day or as needed.

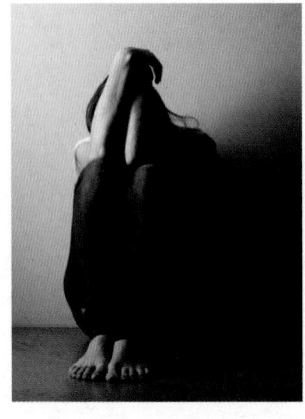

#1 Aurum met: suicidal with despair, worsens at night; extreme insomnia. Only bright sunny day will lift spirits; forms strong attachments with people; suffers in silence, wants no consolation. Symptoms can include heartache, reminiscing, sighing with grief. Can be a "very proper person." May need Natrum mur as well.

#2 Natrum mur: sentimental with flatness, can display watery eyes when in a vulnerable spot, when feeling grief or loss; sighing. "I've already worked it out." Useful when person denies depression, suffers in silence with no consolation.

Alumina: constipated, confused. For depression in the elderly.

Ammonium carb: timid, sad, morose, apprehensive, anxious. Nightmares, intellectual impairment, and ill humor in the morning.

Anacardium: triad of depression, anger, and conflict. Strong inclination to violence.

Calc carb: work-related, can't bear the burdens (see Nat sulph). Feelings of being weighed down, in despair.

Cimicifuga: feeling of black cloud overhead, can think they are crazy. Oversensitive to noise, sleeplessness; symptoms worse in cold, better in warmth and fresh air.

Hypericum: depression from injury to the nerves, from an emotional shock, big trauma. Fear of surgery, anxious and sensitive to movement. Symptoms better in cold, worse after sleeping. Hyper-sensitive to touch.

Ignatia: in conflict, confused, disappointed. Person can often be a perfectionist.

Kali brom: severe depression with blank look, almost immobile or unresponsive; person sits and stares at the wall.

Lachesis: hormonal depression, high blood pressure, self-pity. Person is talkative.

Lycopodium: angry, poor confidence, digestive problems.

Natrum carb: depressed about the state of the world, the levels of suffering. Digestive problems, blues, gloom, melancholy.

Natrum sulph: severely depressed, suicidal, must restrain themselves. Can be from liver problems, overwork, head injury, conflict over who's going to take care of them. Weariness, worse in winter.

Phosphoric acid: triad of depression, apathy, and low energy.

Platinum metallicum: arrogant attitude with masked depression: pride, insulting, as if everything and everyone seems smaller or less significant. Can experience high joyousness, then feel dead lowness; often brought down by small setbacks. Has big ego, high sex drive.

Pulsatilla: hormonal triad of self-pity, sadness, and loneliness; strong need to express while weeping. Needs consolation, sitting at home with a "please-hug-me" look.

Sepia: angry, yelling, wants to be alone; result of estrogen dominance (from pill or childbirth or menopausal hormone fluctuations). Resigned, frustrated, anxious women; worse in cloudy weather. Feels better by movement, exercise.

Silicea: weakness of the mind; lacking grit.

Staphysagria: grief; puts self down: thinks they will never amount to anything. Won't talk; triad of worthlessness, guilt, and depression.

Thuja: feels like a bad person, alien, that no one understands. Feels that they are different, strange, or weird.

Depression States Homeopathy

Lack of Energy

Anacardium: with anger and violence.

Kali phos: for nervous states.

Phosphoric acid: from the loss of loved one, apathy.

Depression from Anguish

Hyoscyamus: with sexual overtones.

Ignatia: with nervousness or from grief.

Passiflora: to ease nervous tension.

Stramonium: from fears and results of violence.

Valeriana: to calm nervous tension.

Depression from Sleep Disorders

Passiflora: used to ease nervous tension.

Valeriana: high and low emotions.

Depression in Adults

Picric acid: where there is memory loss accompanying depression.

Functional Depression (person can work despite being depressed)

Aurum met: suicidal depression in business people or those experiencing financial difficulty.

Natrum mu: grief, isolation, can't be consoled, won't cry in public.

Depression and Anxiety Cell Salts

Depression with the following:

Calc fluor: financial problems.

Calc phos: in children, overstimulation, on waking.

Calc sulph: at night.

Ferr phos: at night, during menses.

Kali phos: at night, overstimulation, in the morning, on waking.

Kali sulph: at night, in the morning.

Mag phos: in the morning.

Nat mur: causeless depression, disappointment, at night, in children, overstimulation, financial loss, menopause, during menses.

Nat sulph: causeless, at night, in the morning, in children.

Silicea: in the morning.

Anxiety with the following:

Calc fluor: money problems.

Calc phos: in the chest, moaning, pain.

Calc sulph: in the chest, at night, in bed, fear, heart palpitations.

Ferr phos: in the chest, at night.

Kali phos: weak nervous system, in the chest, eating, at night, in bed, fear, heart palpitations.

Kali sulph: open air, in the chest, at night, in bed, heart palpitations.

Nat mur: in the chest, at night, in bed, fear, heart palpitations, moaning.

Nat phos: with business, at night, fear, heart palpitations.

Nat sulph: in the chest, in bed.

Silicea: with asthma, in the chest, at night, in bed, fear, heart palpitations, moaning, pain, vertigo.

Depression References

Books

Emotional Healing with Homeopathy
by Peter Chappell

Books by David R. Card

Homeopathy for Today
12 Essential Minerals for Cellular Health
Seven Symbols of Healing

DavesHealingNotes.com

Anger	*Depression*	*Nervousness*
Anxiety	*Memory*	*OCD*
Avoiding eye contact	*Alzheimer's*	*Stress*
Bipolar	*Dementia*	

The Spine

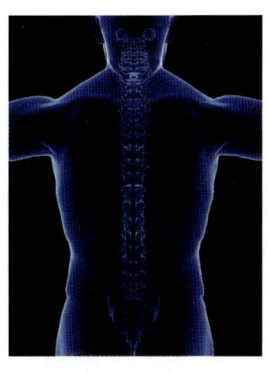

Many herbalists, homeopaths, and other alternative practitioners have watched the spine heal, with results varying from very slight improvement to complete recovery. We don't intend on giving recommendations for all the alternative healing possibilities, but are presenting herbal, homeopathic, and cell salts as supplements. Most natural therapies are gentle and will not interfere or interact with other medicines. Opportunities for healing might include chiropractic care, energy work, massage therapy, acupressure, acupuncture, and more.

We will be discussing acute care where there has been a **recent injury** (emergency care). Acute care is useful and brings quick relief. **Old or recurring problems** can find fast relief through natural anti-inflammatories, but lasting results can take up to 24 months. Sometimes results are partial because the damage is too great. **Any relief** is better than dependence on pharmaceutical drugs.

Today, doctors are generally open-minded, so check with them as you use alternative care. If your doctor objects, ask him why. If he doesn't understand or can't explain why, you might consider shopping for a more open-minded doctor.

Modern medicine uses pain killers, physical therapy and surgery for spinal injuries. The results vary greatly. Sometimes the problems get worse. When a person gets caught up in the "system," they are often convinced there is no other course. Pharmaceutical pain relievers mask and suppress the pain while causing damage to the digestive system (i.e., the liver, intestines). Pain relief in the natural arena is accomplished because the body is healing, and there are few side effects as well.

Spine Emotions

The spine gives the body the **proper posture** which shows in our stature. All **inner pressures** show up in our posture. Posture shows our relationship to God, and our self-esteem. It suffers when we can no longer carry life's burdens. In every case it is not only our spine, but **tension of the muscles** that are affected by our inner conflicts.

Tailbone pains show up from disappointment, aggression, fright, reaction, emotional stress, and lack of humility.

Spinal Discs are responsible for our inner posture and serve as a buffer. They capture injuries and develop problems when they are stressed. When we can't take the stress, then pain occurs. One cannot treat the problem without finding the cause. Spiritually, we are forced to reflect on what burdens us with a pressure that is too much for us.

Spine Facial Diagnosis

Head tilted back and abdomen protruded – spinal damage

Head, posterior sloped or flat – frequent spinal diseases

Ear, hardened, rolled ear border – stiff spine

Eyebrow, raised – spinal changes

Nose, horizontal line across the top of the nose

Cheeks, deep vertical lines between the nose and ear on both sides.

Chin, dimple.

Other body signs of spinal issues

Belly button off center, vertical lines underneath

Belly enlarged

Bone pains

Butt appears out of alignment

Feet flat or other foot distortions

Gait, staggering

Hips, uneven

Legs, uneven length

Pelvis, tilted or distorted, unbalanced

Osteoporosis

Postural hunching

Scoliosis

Thumb, stiff

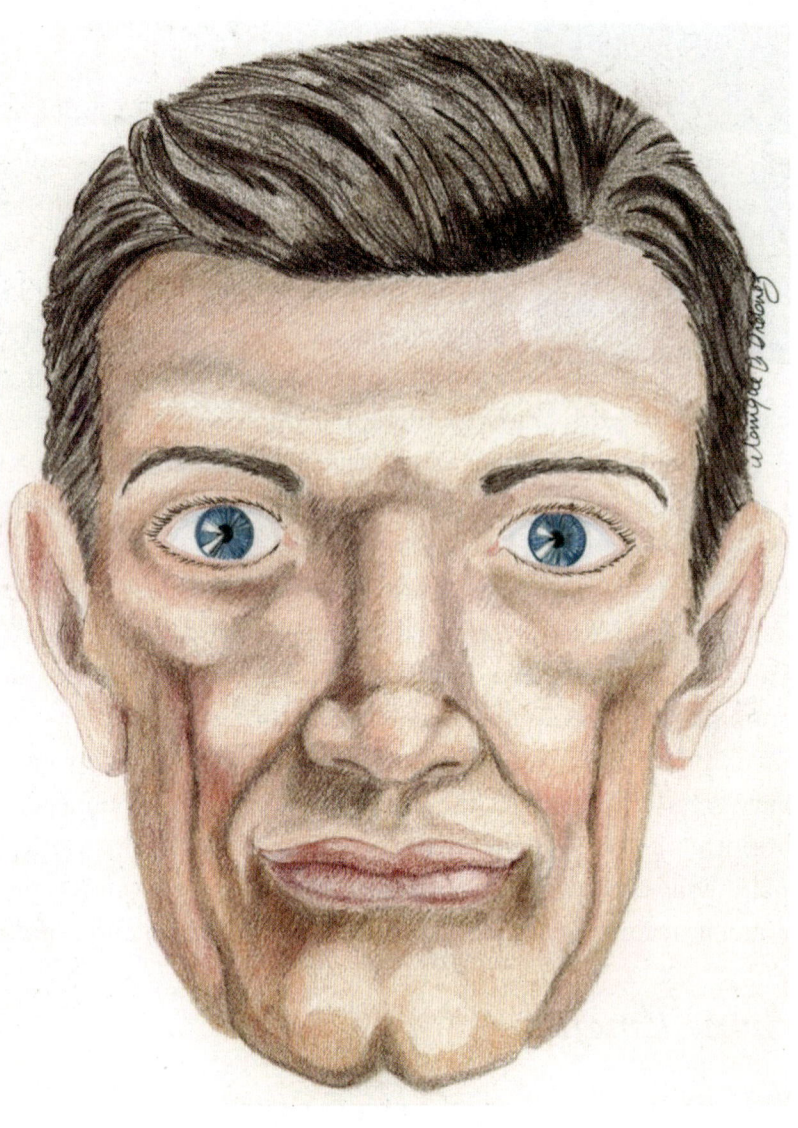

Spine Anti-inflammatory Herbs

Most spices in your kitchen taken on an empty stomach (between meals) can exert an anti-inflammatory effect. Be sure to try the herbs one at a time. You might want to put them in capsules and try one capsule at a time and increase as needed. Some herbs can interfere with medications, but generally don't. If in doubt, consult with your doctor. The following herbs are researched for their anti-inflammatory activities:

Bromelain is a pineapple enzyme capable of pain relief.

Boswellia has anti-inflammatory properties with the side effect of lowering blood pressure.

Cayenne equalizes blood pressure and circulation, and relieves pain.

Celery seed controls gout and relieves pain.

Ginger facilitates better digestion and is anti-inflammatory.

Nettles are good for allergies and are rich in minerals.

Papaya is good for digestion and inflammation.

Peppermint aids digestion and decreases inflammation.

Spearmint has the same properties as peppermint.

Thyme is drying and anti-inflammatory.

Turmeric is a powerful anti-inflammatory.

Valerian is calming and sedating.

Willow contains aspirin-like compounds that are anti-inflammatory.

Yucca has cortisone-like compounds that act powerfully on joints.

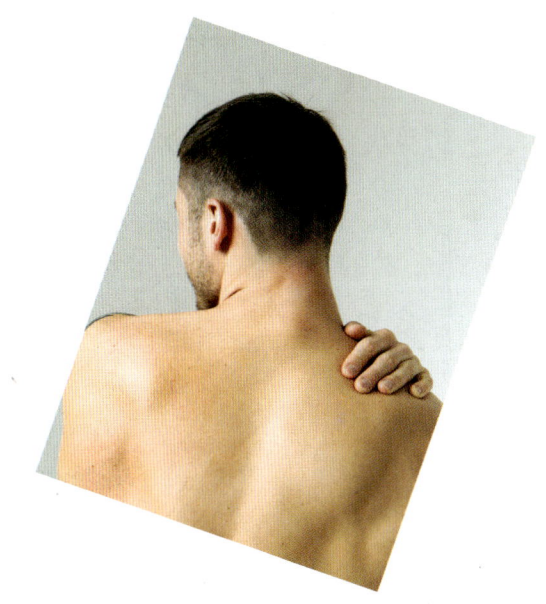

Spine Homeopathic Medicines

Argentum met: splinter pains.

Arsenicum alb: nerve damage, neuralgia.

Calc carb: bone degeneration.

Calc phos: bone building.

Cimicifuga: arthritis, rheumatism, neuralgia.

Cinchona: recovery.

Colocynthis: lumbar pain.

Equisetum: water loss with rheumatism.

Formicum Acid: arthrosis, arthritis, myalgia.

Gelsemium: neuralgia, paralysis, headache.

Hypericum: neuralgia, nerve pinching.

Rhus Tox: rheumatism, neuralgia, neuritis.

Secale: paralysis, spasms.

Sepia: low back with sciatica, mostly women.

Solanum Nigrum: brain circulation.

Strontium Carb: arthritis, spondylitis.

Symphytum: disc repair.

Tabacum: paralysis, neuralgia.

Spine References

Books

Homeopathy for Musculoskeletal Healing
by Asa Hershoff N.D., D.C.

The Homeopathic Emergency Guide
by Thomas Kruzel N.D.

Books by David R. Card:

Facial Diagnosis of Cell Salt Deficiencies
Seven Symbols of Healing

DavesHealingNotes.com

Arthritis, gouty	*Muscle Cramps*	*Sciatic pain*
Arthritis, osteo	*Muscular Dystrophy*	*Spasmodic torticollis*
Arthritis, rheumatoid	*Pain*	*Wry neck*
Bursitis	*Restless Legs*	

Spine Cell Salts

Calc fluor: spinal curvature, disc problems (degeneration, prolapse). For aching, restlessness, and chronic lumbago with strain. Back pains better from motion, warmth, and continued motion, worse from started motion. Burning pain in lower back.

Calc phos: lower back soreness. Sacroiliac feels broken. Back pain with tingling or numbness. Sensitive to movement. Spinal curvature, partial disc prolapse.

Ferrum phos: the top anti-inflammatory. Neck stiffness to upper back with sharp pains. Heat in spots on back. Muscle strain. Partial disc prolapse.

Kali phos: irritated spine with a creeping sensation along with intense pain. Paralytic lameness of the back. Spinal disc degeneration.

Mag phos: cramping pains of the back with stiffness, soreness. Aching of the small of the back. Shooting pains. Sensitive to movement.

Nat mur: needs firm support of the back, feels bruised. Back is worse in the morning, coughing. Better from lying on back and firm pressure. Neck stiff; disc problems. For regeneration after injuries.

Nat phos: back feels heavy. Spinal arthritis. Back feels weak after sex. Nerve damage. Top remedy for lumbago, disc prolapse. Nerve damage, sensitive to movement.

Silicea: spinal weakness, tailbone pain; sensitive after injury, decay of vertebrae. Stiffness of neck with headache, burning sensation, lame sacroiliac joint. Back sore after long car rides. Nerve damage, sensitive to movement. Sensitivity to drafts.

To use these formulas, put required amounts of pellets in a water bottle and sip all day.

Back Support formula
10-Ferrum phos 6X
20-Mag phos 6X
10-Silicea 6X

Spinal Disc Regeneration formula
15-Calc fluor 6X
10-Nat mur 6X
20-Silicea 6X

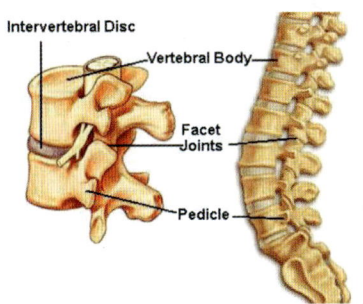

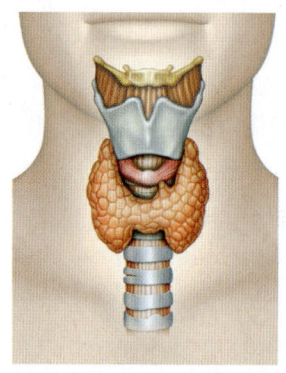

The Thyroid: Hyperthyroid and Hypothyroid

The thyroid is a small gland at the bottom-front of the neck that controls the metabolism of the body, including temperature and energy output. It works with the rest of the endocrine glands including the pituitary, hypothalamus, and adrenals.

Thyroid Emotions

Anonymous Author

Negative:	**Positive:**
Mood swings	Comfortable
Confused thinking	Friendship
Contradictory	Patient
Argumentative	Noble
Demanding	Pleasant
Repulsive	Agreeable
Ridiculing	Witty
Over-emotional	

> "The universe doesn't give you what you want in your mind; it gives you what you demand with your actions."
>
> Steve Maraboli,
> *Unapologetically You: Reflections on Life and the Human Experience*

Hyperthyroid

Hyperthyroid is a sign of a failing thyroid, where the pituitary is releasing TSH to compensate, and the thyroid is enlarging. Symptoms can be painful with fever, sluggishness, and aching muscles. There may be a fluid filled tumor or nodule—a noncancerous hard lump on thyroid. If too large, the gland can be unsightly and can cause hoarseness, difficulty swallowing, and discomfort.

Hyperthyroid can be hereditary and indicates thyroid weakness to some degree. It is more common in women, ages 20 – 40. Often, the onset is seen in the beginning of pregnancy. Auto-antibodies take over the pituitary function. Hyperthyroid can be caused from an infection as well.

Hyperthyroid symptoms and signs:

- In the beginning, not tender, not uncomfortable
- Excess sweating
- Diarrhea
- Eyes look larger or protrude; dry, inflamed. May see double, rarely optic neuropathy
- Eyes seem as if staring, eyelid retracted, 'bug eyes'
- Fatigue

- Goiter (enlarged thyroid)
- Hair loss
- Hands shake: tremor
- Heart palpitations (rapid heartbeat)
- Heat intolerance
- High perspiration; dislike hot weather
- Increased appetite
- Loose bowels and more frequent bowel movement
- Lump sensation upon swallowing
- Male breasts may become enlarged
- Menstrual cycle changes: lighter flow, shorter length of cycle, or lack of menses
- Muscle weakness upper arms, thighs; worse carrying heavy packages, climbing stairs
- Nail margin irregularity; trouble keeping nails clean; nail-bed separation
- Neck enlargement
- Nervous, jumpy, irritable, quarrelsome
- Personality changes
- Pulse quickens, rapid heart palpitations that come and go
- Skin becomes thin, delicate; hair loss
- Skin drying
- Skin can become lumpy, reddish, thick
- Tremors
- Weakness
- Weight loss

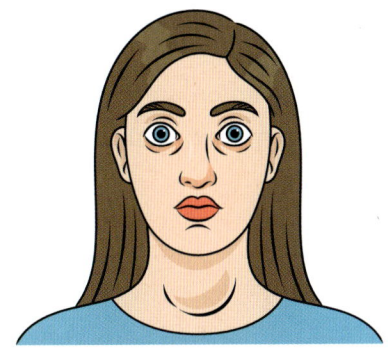

Example:
Grave's Disease - Goiter

Thyroid Cell Salts

- All of the calcium salts (**Calc fluor, Calc phos, Calc sulph**) are important for thyroid health.
- **Ferr phos** is used for inflammation and heat conditions.
- Potassium salts (**Kali mur, Kali phos, Kali sulph**) are important for thyroid health.
- All of the sodiums (**Nat mur, Nat phos, Nat sulph**) are important to the thyroid. **Nat mur** is one of the most important salts for thyroid health and is the one for goiters, thyroid inflammation and hyper or hypothyroid conditions.
- **Mag phos** can be used to support the heart muscle and cramping conditions.
- **Silicea** also plays a part, a general support for thyroid.

Hyperthyroid Facial Diagnosis

Looks younger than they are due to tightness of the skin

Moist forehead and cheek skin in older people

Hair, early graying

Hair loss in women

Long fine eyelashes

Eyes shiny

Eyes too large or "bug out"

Can have an enlarged thyroid as seen when looking up

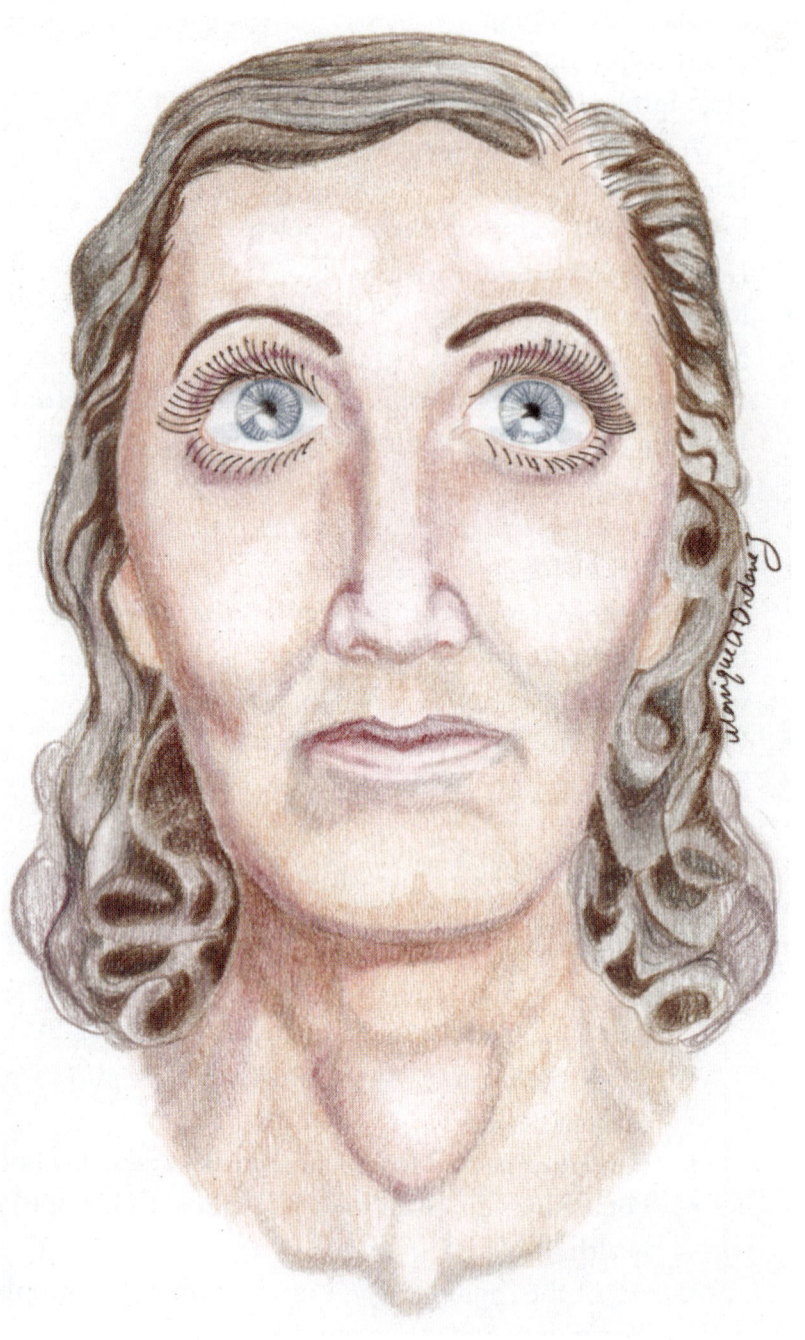

Hyperthyroid (Graves' disease) Herbs

These herbs serve to normalize thyroid function, calm the heart, and reduce stress. This formula for Graves' disease seems to work for most people. Combine 25 drops of each, use it three times a day:

Bugleweed supports the thyroid, helps with heart palpitations.

Motherwort is beneficial for heart palpitations, useful for female hormone levels.

Lemon balm reduces stress, improves digestion, controls heart palpitations, supports the thyroid.

Hyperthyroid Homeopathic Medicines

#1 Iodium: hyperthyroid and goiter, right-sided constriction. Feels hot but dislikes heat. Huge appetite with emaciation, restless, palpitations, pulsations in fingertips.

Belladonna: thyroid swollen, painful, throbbing. High blood pressure, restless, overexcited, and angry.

Cactus: painful with constriction in thyroid and chest; strong palpitations.

Calc carb: hard thyroid and nodules. Feels dull, tired, sluggish; cold hands and feet, internal tremors.

Ferrum met: noise oversensitivity, chest oppression, left-sided goiter. Pale or flushing face. Anemia.

Ferrum iod: obese, goiter from suppressed menses. High blood pressure; pressure on throat. Craves salty fish.

Fluoricum acid: feels hot; worsened by heat. Bone problems, ulcers, varicose veins.

Glonoinum: sun headaches, head feels heavy, strong heart palpitations, throbbing temples, choking sensation, confusion, vertigo.

Natrum mur: disappointed love or grief. Trembling of head, worse from heat or sun. Heart palpitations, nervous, restless.

Phosphorus: right-sided goiter, sensitive. Heart palpitations. Worsened by lying on left side. Intolerant of overstimulation.

Spongia: hard, painful, swollen; choking sensation. Strong heart palpitations, chest feels heavy.

Thyroidinum: feelings of fainting; obesity or emaciation; heart palpitations. Depression upon waking; quarrelsome, not to be contradicted.

Hyperthyroid Cell Salts

Nat mur: with chronic sore throat.

Goiter (Enlarged Thyroid) Herbs

Bladderwrack is rich in iodine for thyroid support.

Kelp is rich in iodine

Poke root is used when there is enlargement of lymph glands.

Thuja is a strong tasting herb used for goiter that also helps with prostate enlargement.

Goiter Homeopathics

Calcarea carb: benign goiter. Obesity. Hypo- or hyperthyroid. Goiter hard with nodules; may be vascular. Slow constant goiter growth. Sweaty head, esp. at night. Internal tremors. When overwork and stress are causes. Tired, slow, cold hands and feet.

Iodium: Hyperthyroid. Right-sided, painful, constricting goiter. Feels hot, emaciation, heart palpitations. Thyroid enlarges, so testes or breasts shrink. Pulsations in fingertips. Hyperactive, restless, great appetite yet loses weight. Can't sit still. Talks incessantly. Intolerance to heat.

Nat mur: thyroid inflammation, hyper or hypothyroid. Emaciation, dryness of lips, heart palpitations. May be caused by grief or disappointed love. Intolerance to heat or sun. Head and/or body trembles. Slow growth and development in children. Likes to be alone. Holds old griefs inside.

Spongia: hard, swollen, painful goiter. Hard to swallow, sharp pains. Suffocating feeling, can't wear tight clothes. Thyroid feels "alive." Hot flashes esp. at night. Chest anxiety, palpitations, and pressure. Testicular inflammation or ovarian pains. Often accompanied with asthma. Can be associated with coughs.

Goiter Cell Salts

Calc fluor: hardness of goiter.

Ferr phos: with inflammation.

Kali sulph: with hoarseness.

Mag phos: hard to swallow.

Nat mur: with chronic sore throat, grief, hoarseness, exhaustion from overactivity.

Nat phos: with pressure sensation.

Nat sulph: with lump sensation in the throat.

Silicea: right-sided goiter; shy, cold person.

Hyperthyroid References

Books

2014 Medicines from the Earth Lecture notes by Jason Miller;

12 Essential Minerals for Cellular Health by David R. Card

DavesHealingNotes.com
Hyperthyroid

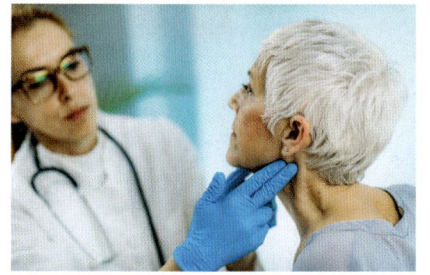

Hypothyroidism

The thyroid is an endocrine gland that controls the body's metabolism through its hormones, along with signals from the pituitary and hypothalamus. The interchange of hormonal signals includes the adrenal glands.

The endocrine system is also influenced by sex hormones, which is evident by the fact that most people who have hypothyroid (low functioning thyroid) are females. Estrogen dominance often influences the thyroid. Modern medicine may create this disease with birth control pills or other drugs that interfere with the estrogen receptors. It can happen after childbirth or sometimes a couple of years into menopause, due to hormonal shifts.

Causes of Hypothyroid

- Iodine deficiency

- In children who never developed enough glandular tissue or who received an inherited defect. Or from too much iodine during mother's pregnancy.

- Children and adults – Hashimoto's or chronic lymphocytic thyroiditis: the most common cause of thyroid failure

- Inflammation and scarring damage

- Can be caused by medical treatment for hyperthyroid

- Temporary failure from viral infection

- Lithium therapy or ingestion

- X-ray therapy in neck area

- Medical treatments that use dye

Pituitary issues related to Hypothyroidism: The pituitary gland controls the thyroid, reproduction and adrenals. Pituitary defects can cause women to stop menstruating. The pituitary is controlled by the hypothalamus.

Signs of Low Thyroid:

- Apathy
- Brittle nails
- Cold intolerance
- Constipation
- Dry hair and skin
- Fatigue
- Forgetfulness
- Goiter
- Hoarseness
- Low blood pressure
- Low voice
- Menstrual changes
- Paleness without anemia
- PMS
- Slowed deep-tendon reflexes
- Stiff, achy, cramping muscles
- Swelling of tissues
- Weakness
- Weight gain

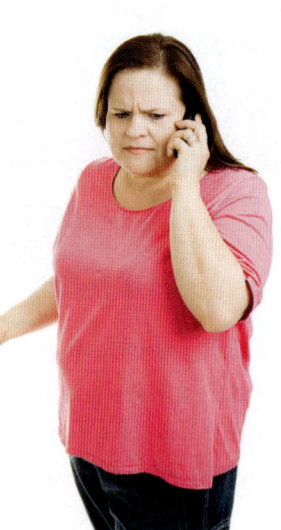

Hypothyroid is a slow process to reverse, but it can happen. The body must have the time and the tools to repair itself. Low functioning of the thyroid may also be connected with an auto-immune disease called Hashimoto's which is failure to produce enough thyroid hormone. High TSH levels portend thyroid failure—the thyroid is trying to compensate.

More serious signs of hypothyroid include:

- Circulation affected, heart rate slows (below 60 beats)
- Intestinal activity slows down (constipation)
- Loss of balance
- Memory loss
- Menses longer, heavier, more frequent
- Muscles sore, swollen, cramping
- Pregnancy difficulties, miscarriage more likely
- Puffy, swollen appearance in face and eyes
- Sensitive to medications
- Tingling in fingers
- Water retention

Hypothyroid References

Books

2014 Medicines from the Earth lecture notes: "The Thyroid" by Jason Miller pg. 180;

12 Essential Minerals for Cellular Health by David R. Card

DavesHealingNotes.com
Hypothyroid

Hypothyroid Facial Diagnosis

High forehead with thin brittle hair

Eyebrows, half are gone

Eyelid drooping and swelling in menopausal women

Eye, border of cornea is opaque

Eyes, squinting ("Eskimo eyes")

Eyes, spider veins on outside of corners

Nose, horizontal lines on the root of nose

Cheeks are light yellow, swollen

Cheeks, face, dry

Cheeks, waxy pale appearance

Lips bluish

Lower half of face is broader than upper half

Expression flattened

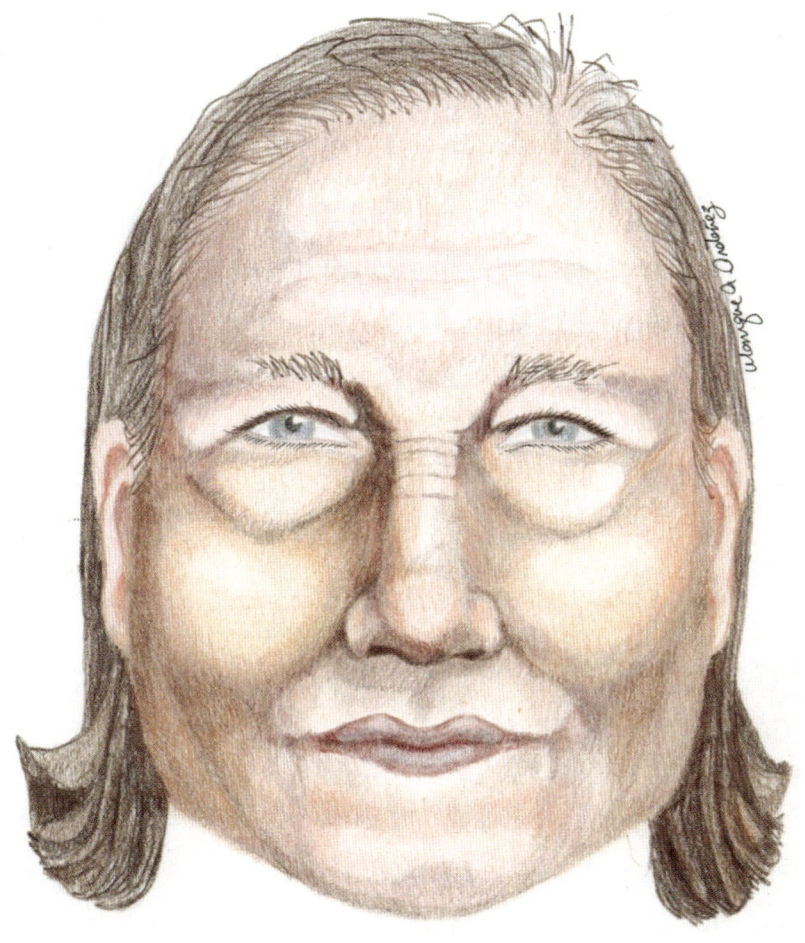

Hypothyroid Supplements

Zinc for immune function – 50 mg per day
Tyrosine for direct thyroid support – 500 mg twice a day on an empty stomach.

Hypothyroid Herbs

It often takes a combination of several herbs to help normalize thyroid function. The strategy is to address adrenal function and help reverse Hashimoto's; stimulate the thyroid into normal hormone production; support the body's iodine stores.

Bladderwrack or **Kelp**, 2 capsules a day to support the iodine supply.

Ashwagandha doubles as an immune normalizer and thyroid stimulant, and an endocrine adaptogen.

Guggul as a thyroid stimulant and normalizer of cholesterol levels.

Eleutherococcus is an adaptogen that supports the endocrine and immune systems.

Hypothyroid Homeopathic Protocols

Use one of the following protocols from Dr. Robin Murphy, N.D.:

Thyroid Protocol I-Hypothyroid
Low thyroid but using no medications: Use one general thyroid remedy: Calcarea carb, Sepia, Natrum mur, or Lycopodium. Stimulates circulation, metabolism, and normalizes thyroid.

Thyroid Protocol II-Hypothyroid
Low thyroid using prescription medications (when have been used for many years): Use most indicated of these remedies: Calcarea carb, Sepia, Natrum mur, or Lycopodium, use for 1-2 months (in 50-60% of people thyroid kicks in); if seeing improvement in 1-2 months, then can be weaned off medication slowly under doctor's supervision.

Coming off thyroid medication "cold turkey" is NOT recommended, but for those who have already done it: Sepia, Calc Carb, Nat Mur, Lycopodium: use in low potency 6c. People often "crash" in 2 weeks or less; if so, then use acute remedy Thyroid 3x or 6x-stop general remedy or give together. Use thyroid remedies first thing in the morning. If thyroid kicks in, the person starts getting warm blooded and restless, which is a good sign!

Thyroid Protocol III-Hypothyroid
Thyroid is atrophied, prescription thyroid medications are not working any more: Use Thyroid 3x or 6x, thyroid massage, thyroid tapping, or eat seaweed or kelp (can be taken in capsules or tablets). Then go to general thyroid remedies in 6c (Calc carb, Nat mur, Lycopodium, Sepia).

In Radioactive iodine damage, there may be a small part still functioning. The cure is in the general above remedies (Calcarea carb, Sepia, Natrum mur, or Lycopodium).

Hypothyroid Homeopathic Medicines

#1 Sepia: cold hands and feet, weight gain, shortness of breath. Craves sweets, exhausted easily, menstrual problems and low sex drive. Yellow skin. Indifference, weeping irritable, sluggish.

#2 Calcarea carb: leg and foot cramps, cold and clammy feet, tendency to gain and lose weight easily, craves sweets. Internal tremor. Head night-sweats. Depression, worry.

Alumina: extreme constipation or soft stools. Thick, dry, itching skin. Slow physically and mentally.

Argentum nit: hot, worsens in warm rooms, fears, hurried feelings, diarrhea, gas, tremors.

Calc iod: hormonal problems, big appetite, worsens in hot rooms, emaciated, heart palpitations, anxiety felt in chest.

Conium: hard goiter. Weakness of thighs, feels cold, heat flushes, weakness, fatigue, cross-eyed, photophobia, dizzy.

Gelsemium: weakness, sleepy, weak and shaky inside, double vision. Droopy eyelids. Fear of the future.

Graphites: chilly, worsens with heat, obesity, fatigue, body pulsations, thick cracking skin, coarse hair.

Kali carb: chilly, sensitive to drafts, constipation, overworking, pains in back.

Kali iod: worsens with heat, allergies, mucus congestion, hurried and irritable or fun and amusing.

Lycopodium: right sided. Can't skip meals, can't take pressure.

Natrum mur: caused by grief or disappointed love. Intolerance to sun or heat. Trembling of body or head. Violent heart palpitations.

Nux vomica: digestive problems, chilly, overheated, trembling; tense, hurried, irritable.

Spongia tosta: swollen hot painful goiter. Swelling and stitching throat pains. Violent palpitations. Chest pressure, suffocative sensation. May also have asthma.

Thyroidinum: sleepy and tired, faints upon standing. Tremors. May be either obese or emaciated.

Hypothyroid Cell Salts

Calc phos: with hoarseness, hurts to swallow.

Nat mur: with lump in throat sensation. Goiter with sore throat, worsens with grief.

Silicea: enlarged thyroid. Right side swollen, affecting swallowing.

The Heart

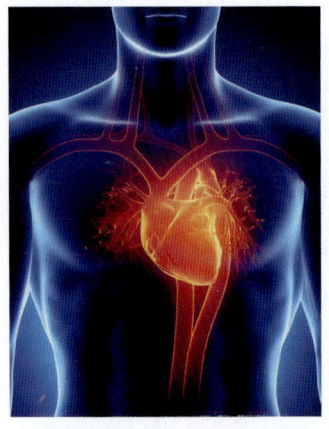

The heart pumps blood which carries oxygen and nourishment to every part of our body. It is essential to life as we know it. Heart health is affected by our dietary habits, vices, the way we move, and our emotions. The human heart beats 60 to 90 times a minute at rest.

Common issues facing those with heart problems are: high blood pressures, valve problems, heart enlargement, arrhythmias, heart attacks, and more.

Exercise temporarily raises your heart rate, but will lower the resting heart rate in the long term, and is good for heart health.

High blood pressure is defined by systolic (the first number) and diastolic (the second number). The numbers are:

- Borderline: 120-140/90-94
- Mild: 140-160/95-104
- Moderate: 140-180/105-144
- Severe: 160+/115+

High blood pressure may come from stress, a diet rich in animal fats, and toxicity related to use of tobacco, alcohol, coffee and tea. I believe most high blood pressure issues are from financial stress. The way we value ourselves and others can have correspondences with heart health. In most cases of high blood pressure the cause is a great mystery, according to the modern health perspective.

Heart and Its Role

The heart is the center of our existence; it houses our feelings, especially love, and is the area of emotional understanding. Heart procedures and medications can affect how we think and how we feel, because whatever affects the heart affects our emotions. Many people change their outlook on life, as well as experience emotional changes, from having heart issues.

The heart is the engine of our body, and has no rest as long as we live. When our heart rhythm is off, it may be a sign that the rhythm of our life is disturbed. The sickest people are ones that only consult their head, and not their heart. Tightness of chest may indicate angina, a feeling of narrowness of the chest, which may also indicate too much ego involvement.

There are many sayings in our society about the heart. In addition to the following, what are some of the sayings you use?

- The heart is the center of feeling and the seat of love
- I have lost my heart
- Heartless person
- Heartfelt thanks
- Follow your heart
- Broken heart
- Do it whole-heartedly
- Hard hearted
- I feel my heart in my throat
- He wears his heart on his sleeve
- Oh, my heart
- Home is where the heart is

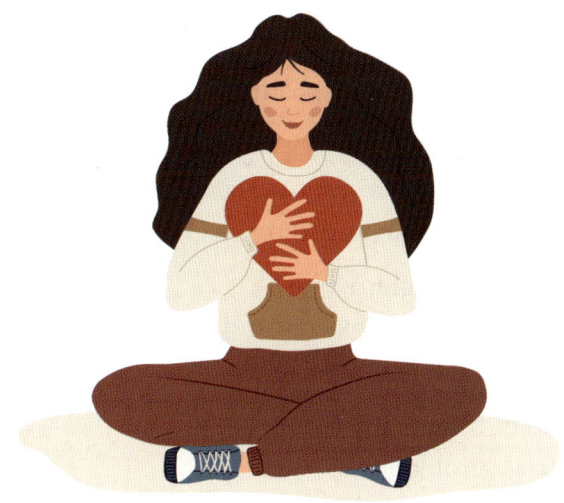

Heart Emotions

Anonymous Author

Negative:	**Positive:**
Lack of emotion	Forgiveness
Talkative	Compassion
Anxious	Love
Hate	Feeling secure
Self-doubt	Thoughtfulness
Unstable	Self-worth
Distrust	Generosity
Bears grudges	Delight
Abusive	Kindness

"The best and most beautiful things in the world cannot be seen or even touched. They must be felt with the heart."

– Helen Keller

Heart Facial Diagnosis

Forehead, lip, cheek, earlobe bluish color – heart insufficiency or low stomach acid

Temples have blue snake-like veins – right heart insufficiency

Earlobes shrunken – disposition to heart attack

Earlobes, knot where ear connects to the head – left heart problems

Face bluish with shiny blue lips – central lack of oxygen and circulation

Face violet blue – heart-lung circulatory problems

Face red – disposition to heart attack

Dull appearance of eyes

Upper eyelids swollen, blue – heart insufficiency

Eye bags hanging – disposition to heart attack

Eye bags swollen and waxy – heart insufficiency

Lower eyelid soreness – heart circulatory disturbance

Milky brown paleness of face – inflammation in lining of the heart (endocarditis)

Left cheek drooping (image is reversed)

Cheeks reddish blue with a pale nose and chin

Lengthened naso-labial lines from nose to corner of mouth

Short nose – disposition to heart failure

Root of nose small – nervous heart condition

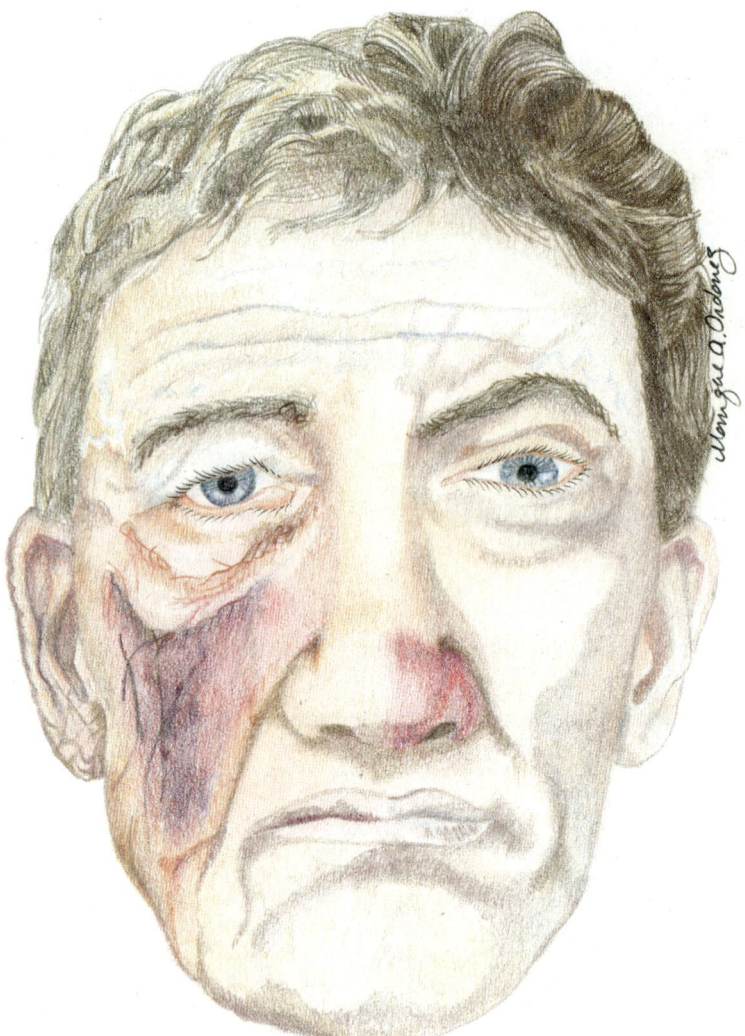

Red nose enlarged with varicose veins – heart disturbances

Nostrils bluish red

Lips bluish or violet, with overall paleness – heart insufficiency

Tongue tip red – heart congestion

Tongue blue-purple – collapse symptoms

Tongue, crack down center to the tip

Chin and lower lip numbness – old heart attack

Neck, shortened – disposition to heart disturbances

Neck with blue stripes – advanced heart changes

Heart Herbs

Heart herbs, taken individually or in combination, can improve overall heart health. Combinations usually work best unless there is a specific condition.

Cayenne normalizes blood pressure and equalizes circulation. It has been known to stop bleeding and heart attacks.

Garlic, fresh or prepared any other way is universally acceptable for heart health. It is non-toxic and helps with high blood pressure and cholesterol.

Hawthorn leaves, flowers, and **berries** have been shown to reduce blood pressure and tone up all the heart functions. It also helps for sleep.

Lemon Balm is often combined with hawthorn as a heart tonic and a nervine relaxant.

Linden Flowers are a cardio tonic as well as reducing the blood pressure. It is a natural anti-inflammatory. It works on the heart through the nervous system.

Motherwort is a nervine, antispasmodic, and lowers high blood pressure. It is especially good for heart palpitations. It is also used to help menstrual disorders.

Valerian is usually known to calm down the nervous system and improve sleep. It also calms the heart.

Yarrow is another cardiovascular tonic that tones the blood vessels, reduces high blood pressure. It also reduces excess menstrual bleeding.

Diuretics are often used to reduce blood pressure, to aid the kidneys to remove excess water. One of the best diuretic herbs is **Shave grass** as it stimulates the kidneys. Other natural diuretics can be used.

Heart Homeopathic Medicines

30c potency can be taken along with prescription medications; combinations may be used as well. Do not go off prescription medications; as symptoms improve with homeopathic medicines, consult your healthcare professional to reduce those medications.

Angina Homeopathic Medicines (for oppression of the chest)

Aconite: angina with panic.

Arnica: from over-exhaustion and numbness; can be useful for strong, earthy persons who don't get easily freaked out.

Glonoinum: heart palpitations so strong, the person next to them can hear it. Carotids (temples) are throbbing.

Spigelia: violent audible palpitations of the heart and severe, shocking or compressive pains. Sensitivity to touch of any part of the body. Heart pains worsen from motion, cold, wet weather.

Heart Attack Homeopathic Medicines

Don't stop your heart medications, always consult your doctor. Diet plays a big part: low meat, low fat, low sugars.

Crotalus hisp: worse lying on the right side; weakness and feels as if the heart turns over in the chest. Dark bruising, parts look bluish, face dark, fingernails blue.

Naja: suicidal feelings, imaginary problems cause brooding. Severe stitching or weakness felt in chest, cramping in left neck and shoulder. Worse lying on left side, better from fresh air.

Spigelia: same as above.

Tabacum: dizziness, weakness, seasickness, vomiting and chilliness with a cold sweat, accompanied by headaches, diarrhea and palpitations. Twisting pain around the heart. Tabacum affects the vagus nerve, which has impact on the stomach and the heart.

Heart Cell Salts

Calc fluor: arteriosclerosis, aneurysm, heart valve hardening, endocardium fibrous deposits.

Ferr phos: first stage cardiovascular problems, inflammation, congestive palpitations.

Mag phos: heart muscle pain (angina), heart constriction sensation, nervous spasms.

Nat mur: fluttering heart sensation, sharp pains, palpitations. Heart enlargement. Weak, vulnerable, from grief. High blood pressure from excess salt intake. Heart cold, empty or constricted-feeling.

Silicea: from nervous exhaustion, throbbing all over the body.

Heart References

Books

Facial Diagnosis of Cell Salt Deficiencies, 12 Essential Minerals for Cellular Health by David R. Card

DavesHealingNotes.com
Blood Pressure

The Lungs

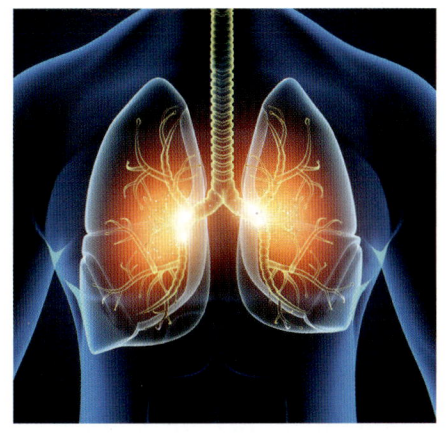

The lungs' job is to provide oxygen for the cells of the body and to get rid of carbon dioxide as a waste product. The alveoli of the lungs exchange the gases and have an average surface area of over one hundred square meters, and this is why the system works well. The lungs represent the heart/lung chakra, where one sees the transition from physical to spiritual circumstances.

Coughs are irritations of the lungs, bronchitis and pleurisy both come from inflammation, asthma brings tightness, and pneumonia comes from infection.

Problems with the lungs are seen by the Chinese as **grief**. The lung hour is around 4 am. Emotional effects of grief and sadness can damage the lungs, along with nervous and stress conditions. It is most apparent in those people born on Wednesdays, or the day of Mercury. Those born in the Mercury or lung hour can also have this risk. Mercury was known as the messenger of the gods. He is often depicted with wings on his helmet and shoes. You can read more about Mercury in my book *Seven Symbols of HEALING*.

Another system representing the zodiac is Gemini (May 22 to June 21), and it governs the lungs. Therefore, those born within this time period are likely affected. Dr. George Carey recommended the regular use of the cell salt Kali mur (potassium chloride) for both those born during this time period and those affected by respiratory problems.

In Chinese medicine we find the lung meridian. Significant lung acupressure points are located on the front of the body just under the shoulders. When these points are sore, there is a lung meridian imbalance which may indicate respiratory problems as well as grief.

For general lung health Chinese medicine recommends a tongue scraper (don't brush your tongue), used at least once a day. This reduces respiratory problems up to 75 percent.

Causes of Lung Problems

Weather – drafts of cold or dry winds or cold dampness that goes deep to the bones.

Geographical locations – high altitude or by the seashore.

Diet and lifestyle – eating foods that cause mucus, primarily dairy products. All people with respiratory problems should avoid dairy, sugar, and processed foods. Also, foods that cause gas can inflate the stomach and put pressure on the lungs and heart.

Lung Emotions
Anonymous Author

Negative:	**Positive:**
Melancholy	Cheerful
Self-pity	Humility
Perplexed	Modesty
Heartache	Openness
False pride	Tolerance
Haughty	Optimistic
Depressed	Unselfish
Intolerance	Meek
Regret	

> "One must absorb the life-giving creative spirit of good, and reject the toxic, deadly and destructive spirit of evil."

Chinese System of Healing – Lawson Wood

Lung References

Books
Homeopathic Therapeutics, Vol III, Diseases of the Ear, Nose, Throat, and Respiratory System
by Prakash Vakil

Books by David R. Card:
Seven Symbols of Healing, Facial Diagnosis of Cell Salt Deficiencies, Homeopathy for Today

DavesHealingNotes.com
Spring Allergies-download
Allergies, food
Allergies, hay fever
Allergies, pet dander
Asthma
Bronchitis
COPD
Emphysema
Flu
Pleurisy
RSV

Lung Facial Diagnosis

Blueness of lips, cheeks, forehead – insufficient oxygen

Redhead

Ears, knot on earlobe of lung affected

Ears blue – chronic bronchitis

Deep lines under the lower eyelids

Cheeks sunken, blue

Cheek redness – weak lungs

Nose blue – asthma, breathing disturbance

Nose, spider veins root at root – lung disease

Nasal entrance distorted – bronchial problems

Nostril opening thickness – diseased or weak lungs

Abnormally wider nose – sign of possible lung disease.

Enlarged nasal passages – breathing difficulties

Nose holes widened (nasal flaring) – bronchial asthma

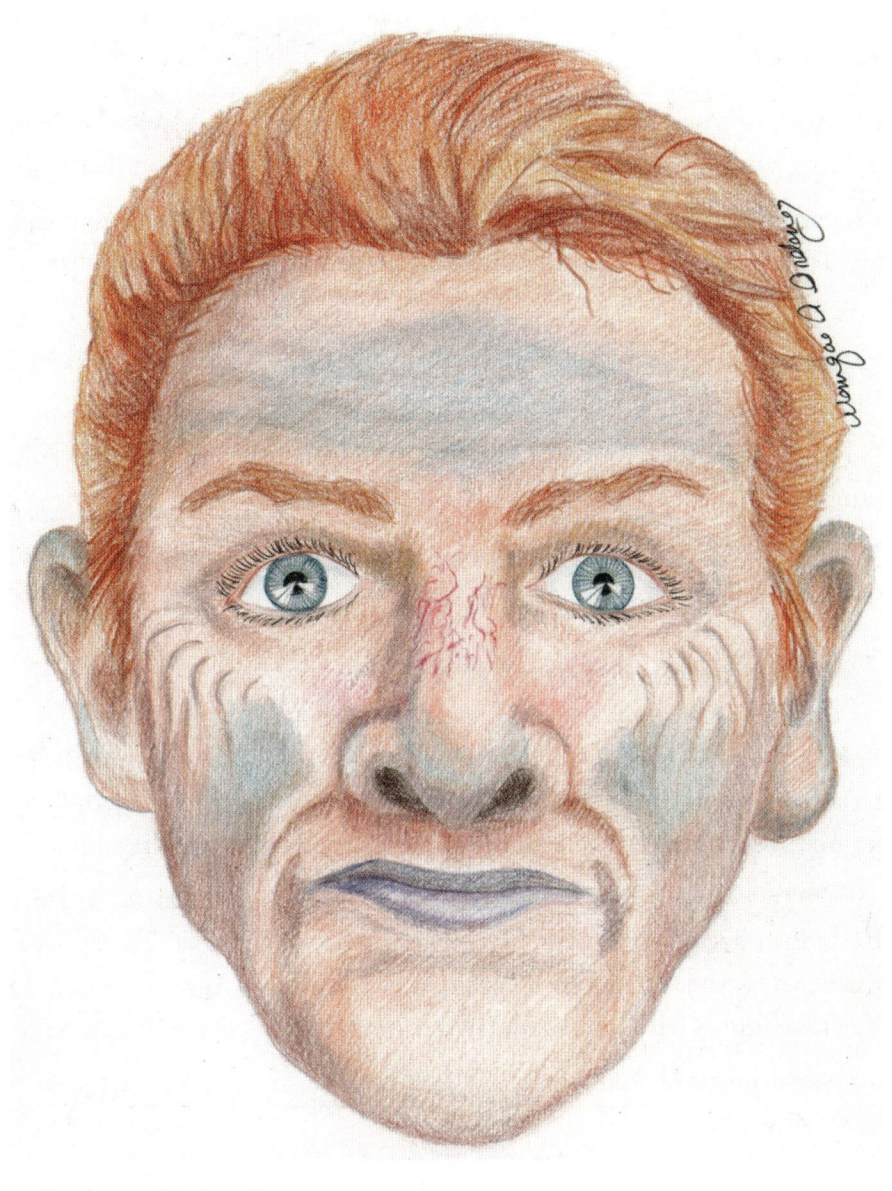

Lung Herbs

Herbs for the lungs relax them (antispasmodic), reduce mucus, and are antimicrobial and anti-congestive.

Catnip improves lungs by reducing mucus and helping with allergies.

Elecampane is a respiratory decongestant that helps by improving digestive function to reduce mucus.

Fenugreek dissolves mucus in the lungs and sinuses and improves digestion.

Garlic is warming and antimicrobial for weak lungs.

Horehound helps to reduce wet coughs by drying mucus and improving digestion.

Licorice soothes the mucus membranes and acts on inflammation along with other herbs.

Lobelia reduces tension on tight lungs for dry coughs, helping to relax the lungs.

Mullein is used for congestion, dry coughs and asthma, as well as for excessive fluids.

Sage is warming, removes excessive mucus and is antimicrobial.

Thyme is warming and improves lung function by reducing mucus.

Lung Homeopathic Medicines

Spongia tosta for cough, hoarseness (dry, scratchy, raw) with foreign sensation in the larynx. Acute and chronic larynx inflammation. Sweating.

Belladonna, Spongia tosta, Hyoscyamus for painful irritating cough, pain and rawness under the breastbone. Medium to high fever. Sweating.

Hyoscyamus and **Aconite** before bed for bronchitis.

Antimonium sulf aur and **Ammonium mur** for painful irritating cough. No fever, whitish yellow mucus, hard to breathe; cause can be change of weather.

Arsenicum album for chronic cough; exhaustion, loss of appetite, weight loss, night sweats, low fevers. Menstrual disturbances. (Looks like lung tuberculosis or possible lung cancer.)

Phosphorus in exchange with **Antimonium tart** for painful cough; chills, high fever that begin quickly. Pains in the sides. After 2 days a rust-colored sputum. Hard to breathe (may look like pneumonia).

Aconite, Antimonium tart for cough, medium fever. After bronchitis, slow onset, hard to breathe. Often in children or aged. Often a complication of an infection (bronchial pneumonia).

Aconite for strong irritable cough; sudden stitching pains on one side of the chest. Loss of breath, pale, restless, anxious, weak pulse, bloody discharge (lung embolism).

Spirea ulmaria mother tincture, **Aconite** and **Bryonia** in exchange, for cough, side pains; painful breathing, slow onset, strong fever. Rib inflammation.

Echinacea drops, Aconite and **Gelsemium** in exchange, for cough with headache, fever, chills; sore throat, heavy disease feeling, influenza. Danger of complication (brain inflammation or pneumonia).

Asthma – Allergy Homeopathic Medicines

Arsenicum album: worse 11 pm to 2 am with restlessness.

Lycopodium: aggravation from 4pm to 8 pm, worse on right side of body, liver problems.

Natrum mur: general allergies with dryness or excess salty clear watery mucus and dry irritated eyes.

Natrum sulph: 4am aggravation, congested liver.

Sulpwhur iod: ears, nose and throat, hot and irritating cough.

Sulphur: feels hot and may have alternating skin problems.

Pneumonia Homeopathic Medicines

Aconite: acute from a cold dry wind; fever present.

Bryonia: hurts to cough, with sharp pains.

Chelidonium: with gallbladder problems, mostly right-sided.

Ferrum phos: low fever, flu onset.

Phosphorus: oversensitive, especially the left lung, tight chest, burning symptoms.

Veratrum viride: with heart involvement.

Homeopathy for Time of Asthma onset

Waking – Alumina, Conium, Sepia

10 am – Carcinosinum

10 – 11 am Ferrum metallicum

Noon – Lobelia

9 pm – Bryonia

10 pm Aralia Racemosa, Mephites

11 pm – Grindelia

11pm – 2 am – ARS ALB, Ars Iod

Midnight – Sambucus, Ars Alb

2 am – ARS ALB, Kali Bic, Med, Rumex

2-3 am KALI ARS, KALI CARB

2-4 am Kali Carb, Med

3 am – Cinchona, Cuprum met, KALI CARB, KALI NIT, Nux Vomica

4-5 am – Kali Sulf, Nat Sulf, Stann

5 am – Kali Iod, Nat Sulf

NWS (Never Well Since) Pneumonia

These remedies are for when one is weakened or sickly as a result of having recovered poorly from pneumonia:

Carbo veg: problems from overheating or cold. Old-persons face in young people.

Kali carb: Infantile pneumonia, swollen eyelids, wheezing, rattling, frequent colds.

Phosphorus: weakness, oversensitivity; chest tightness.

Sulfur: to awaken the immune system, especially after antibiotics.

Bronchitis Homeopathic Medicines

Antimonium tart: chronic in the elderly or children; lots of mucus with no power to expel. Rattling mucus, suffocation, oppression: must sit up. Worse in the morning, evening, when lying down. Vomiting, diarrhea, hopeless, despondent.

Baryta mur: old or young. Suffocation, coughs all night, weight on chest, shortness of breath, chilly in the day, night-sweats with weakness.

Bryonia: dry stitching in chest. Worse at night, with motion.

Drosera: elderly, especially w/emphysema. Worsens with lying down, night, spring and fall. Cough comes from abdomen, yellow mucus.

Ferrum Phos: children; acute, short spasmodic, painful. Worse at night. Pregnancy: cough w/ urine leaking.

Hepar Sulph: rattling chocking; moist; worse in the morning and after eating, and when uncovering body.

Ipecac: children; mucus causing suffocation; worse in moist warm room. Spasms, nausea, vomiting.

Lycopodium: depressing, fatiguing, tickling cough. Worse 4 – 8 pm, during sleep, when stooping, lying down, or eating cold foods and drinks. Dyspepsia.

Phosphorus: chronic, elderly. Cough with tearing pains in chest. Suffocation of upper chest and larynx, panting. Dry short barking cough, stringy mucus; worse evening to midnight, can't lie on left side.

Pulsatilla: lots of thick yellow mucus. Better with cold open air, worse warm room. Must sit up, loss of smell, tongue coated.

Sanguinaria: dry cough at pit of throat; pain in sternum. Teasing dry hacking cough. Constriction, deep breaths, and tearing pain. Painful sighing respiration.

Spongia: croupy, dry, day and night. Hard, dry racking cough; worse hot room, lying; better sitting, eating and drinking.

Silicea: children. Worsens with cold drinks, better moist warm air. Mucus worse lying on back or stooping.

Stannum: hoarse, dry cough where mucus is expelled with great force; copious green sweetish expectoration. Cough excited by laughing, talking, etc.

Tuberculinum: worse in closed room, with motion, when standing, change of weather. Damp, cold drafts 10 pm – 3 am, fear of animals in children. Dry hacking cough, profuse sweating, loss of weight, suffocation.

Lung Cell Salts

Ferr phos: first stage of inflammation, acute bronchial mucus.

Kali mur: thick white mucus, hard to cough up.

Kali phos: whooping cough with yellow mucus.

Kali sulph: rattling mucus in lungs, whooping cough.

Nat mur: sighing from emotional states, suffocation.

Nat sulph: hard to breath in damp weather.

Silicea: shortness of breath, emphysema.

Asthma – Allergy Cell Salts

Calc sulph: with fever, morning, night.

Ferr phos: cough worse morning, evening.

Kali mur: with gastric problems, white mucus.

Kali sulph: coarse cough, slimy yellow mucus.

Mag phos: spastic nervous asthma.

Nat mur: clear salty mucus.

Nat phos: chest pain, cough worse sitting.

Nat sulph: humid asthma, worse damp, worse 4 - 5 am.

Silicea: spasms, worse from drafts, lying down.

Bronchitis Cell Salts

Calc fluor: croup, hoarseness, coughing spasm.

Ferr phos: especially in children.

Kali phos: shortness of breath.

Nat mur: emotional, clear salty mucus.

Nat sulph: egg-white mucus, worse in damp.

Silicea: can't breathe lying on back.

Pneumonia Cell Salts

Calc sulph: late stage, pus, rattling mucus.

Ferr phos: coughing up blood.

Kali mur: with thick white mucus.

Kali sulph: wheezing, rattling mucus.

Nat mur: rattling mucus.

Nat sulph: rattling chest, worse damp/humid.

Silicea: with pus: cold, weak, thin person.

The Kidneys

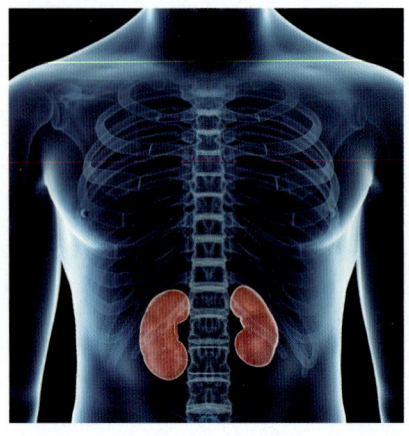

The kidneys are arguably some of the most important organs of the body. The kidneys have the responsibility to filter the blood, clean and detoxify. The responsibility of the kidneys is to be a filtration station; they must determine what is good for the organism and remove what is damaging, what is useless, and what is conflicting.

Chinese medicine characterizes the **kidneys** as the **"mother"** or **foundation of life** as we know it. According to the Chinese it includes the urinary system, sexual functioning, the knees, ears, hair, and teeth. Problems in any of these areas may mean weak or unbalanced kidney function.

Some authors think that kidney problems are a physical sign of **unresolved partner relationships**. Kidney problems arise from conflicts with a partner, especially about sexuality (uterine or prostate issues), and interpersonal relationships in general. (Indeed, all physical problems are connected to emotional or spiritual issues. Some are obvious and some are very subtle.)

Our language also connects us to sayings about our kidneys, which are connected to emotions. For example, "He was so scared that he wet his pants," or "She is all pissed off."

Fears are connected to urinary function. We just have to think about our present or past situation or lifestyle. Our intimate relationships, including sex, also relate to kidney function, the uterus and the prostate. Fear injures the kidneys.

Kidney issues can indicate problems with self esteem. They can also reveal an inability to accept new circumstances, or hanging onto the past. They also can indicate impure thoughts that we keep inside.

The kidneys are responsible for the balance between the **male acidic and the female alkaline** powers and harmony between them. The goal is to find the balance and remove what is no longer needed.

Causes of Kidney Problems

- Antibiotics
- Appendicitis
- Arteriosclerosis
- Bad blood transfusions
- Bronchitis
- Cystitis, Chronic or Severe acute
- Enlarged prostate
- Environmental toxins
- Extensive burns
- High blood pressure
- High Cholesterol
- Inherited Kidney disease
- Injuries
- Kidney Stones
- Medications, over-the-counter drugs and prescriptions
- Pain killers
- Pelvic inflammation
- Pneumonia
- Scarlet fever
- Sinus infections
- Teeth root infections
- X-ray exposure

Important Symptoms of Kidney disease

- Raised blood pressure, esp. diastolic
- Protein in the urine
- Blood in the urine
- Swelling around the eyes
- Low back pain
- Heart problems
- Earaches

Kidney Emotions
Anonymous Author

Negative:	Positive:
Foreboding	Contemplative
Forgetfulness	Decisive
Phobia	Loyal
Superstitious	Cautious
Disloyal	Sexual Security
Uncaring	Stability
Reckless	Inventive
Indecisive	Resolute
Overcautious	Trusting
Sexual Insecurity	Satisfaction

"I learned that courage was not the absence of fear, but the triumph over it. The brave man is not he who does not feel afraid, but he who conquers that fear."

– Nelson Mandela

Kidney Facial Diagnosis

Bloated face

Dirty yellow-gray paleness

Deep lines in forehead

Top of ears malformed or misshapen or flattened

Temples, large snake-like veins over the temples

Skin tags on the upper eyelids in women

Eye area swollen

Eyelids, swelling of the upper eyelids, possibly bluish

Lower eyelids swollen and pale

Eye sacks swollen

Cheeks sunken on both sides

Vertical lines above and below the lips

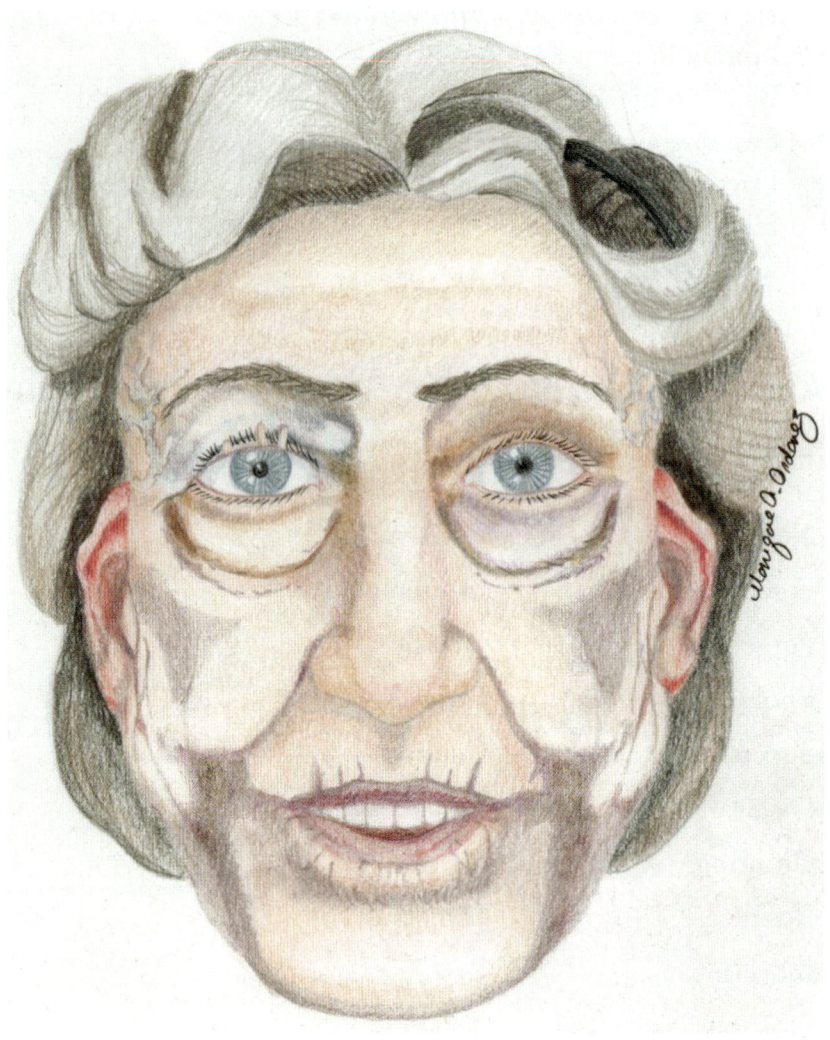

Other Body Signs

Ring fingernail distorted

Fingernail moons are almost gone

Chronic white spots in the fingernails

Headaches start on back of the head and move to the front

Kidney Herbs

> ### Top Herbs for the Kidneys:
> **Astragalus** is a traditional Chinese herb for the kidneys and the immune system in general.
>
> **Dong quai** is a well-used Chinese herb to enrich the blood and promote circulation.
>
> I recommend these two Chinese herbs in combination, as they have been shown to help normalize kidney function.

Chickweed has been used as a poultice after vasectomy, which causes swelling of the testicles.

Cleavers is similar to Corn silk. Males use it for long-term chlamydia; for feeling like kicked in the crotch when lifting light weights. For no pain with scarring in urinary system.

Corn silk, only fresh tincture works best. Potassium sparing, silica rich. UTI from sex. Milder and less irritating than Uva ursi.

Dandelion Leaf in elderly high blood pressure. Better than beta blockers. Useful in congestive heart failure along with hawthorn and cactus. Swelling.

Horsetail is stronger and has more silica. Chronic urinary inflammation with blood in the urine.

Marshmallow is demulcent (soothing) on the genito-urinary tract. Burning cystitis, interstitial cystitis.

Nettle seed is a phenomenal diuretic. Rich in iron and calcium. Prevents and treats osteoporosis. For low-grade kidney pain. For degenerative kidney function. Can help with getting off dialysis if caught in time. Polycystic kidney disease.

Saw Palmetto for treating benign prostatic hypertrophy (BPH). Also for interstitial cystitis, scalding urine.

Kidney Herbs – Diuretics

Buchu has been used for prostate issues, swelling, kidney stones, urinary tract infections; and is stimulating.

Cleavers is for lymphatic swelling and for kidney stones, but not to be used in diabetes.

Garden Carrot is nutritive, tonic, and for kidney stones.

Gravel root is a nervine, used for kidney stones, and genito-urinary problems.

Juniper berry is a stimulating diuretic, good for swelling, the heart and tightness in chest.

Parsley is tonic, antispasmodic, used for kidney stones. Parsley leaf is mild, parsley roots are stronger.

Kidney Herbs – Antibacterial

Blueberries are anti-sticking of bacteria and for stomach H-pylori.

Buchu is an anti-bacterial but less irritating, for nephritis, and acute cystitis.

Cranberries can prevent bacteria from adhering to the lining of the bladder wall (good prevention).

Juniper berry gets rid of uric acid. Irritates the kidneys. Use for only 2 weeks.

Uva ursi is a urinary antiseptic for short term use. Irritating, it inhibits absorption. Used for infections but not with cranberries. Not a diuretic.

Yarrow is for passive blood in urine. Repairs damaged tissues.

Kidney Herbs – Urinary Pain

Agrimony is anti-inflammatory, anti-bacterial, for nervous bladder (like doing Detrol). Post-partum urinary control.

Black Cohosh assists in testicular and renal colic.

Hydrangea is used as a urinary pain reliever and kidney stone dissolver.

Kava is for anxiety and UTI pain. Kidney colic. Interstitial cystitis.

Kidney Homeopathic Medicines

Apocynum can: stimulates urine flow.

Apis mellifica: inflammation of the kidney, uric acid tendency, swelling, inflammation of the mucus membranes.

Berberis vulg: kidney gravel or stones, uric acid tendency, liver function disturbances, rheumatic tendency.

Cantharis: diseases of the kidney, nephritis, prostatitis.

Equisetum: bedwetting, irritable bladder, kidney and bladder stones, uric acid tendency, acute and chronic nephritis, diuretic.

Helleborus: nephritis, hernia, cramps of the bladder musculature, mucus membrane bleeding.

Hypericum: skin problems, nerve problems or damage.

Lycopodium: right sided kidney problems.

Solidago: nephritis, gout, cystitis.

Silicea: constitutional for thin cold delicate shy person; kidney cysts, broken or weak fingernails.

Thuja: cystitis, rheumatic tendency.

Kidney References

Books

Facial Diagnosis of Cell Salt Deficiencies, Seven Symbols of Healing by David R. Card

DavesHealingNotes.com
Bed wetting
Cystitis
Gout
Incontinence
Interstitial cystitis
Kidney stones

Kidney Cell Salts

Calc phos: kidney pain in back, frequent dark urination with strong odor, foam in toilet.

Calc sulph: kidney damage, severe pain, weakening, pus in urine, mucus in urine.

Ferr phos: copious urinating, frequent urge to urinate, bedwetting, incontinence; leaking when coughing. Urinates after every drink.

Kali mur: kidney problems with water retention (edema). Dribbling. Thick mucus in urine. May have diabetes.

Kali phos: bedwetting in nervous children or elderly. Incontinence. Dark yellow urine. Urination comes out in spurts.

Mag phos: bladder nerve pains after a catheter. Sharp pains before urination. Bedwetting in nervous children.

Nat mur: Inability to urinate if other is in room. Very thirsty, gulping. Urinates every hour at night. Leaking while coughing or laughing. Pain after urination.

Nat phos: frequent urination. Waits to start. Needs to urinate after sex with burning, itching.

Nat sulph: frequent copious urination. Burning. Sediment. Gets up frequently at night.

Silicea: profuse urination, foul, thick discharges. Kidney or bladder stones. Bedwetting from parasites.

The Adrenals: Stress

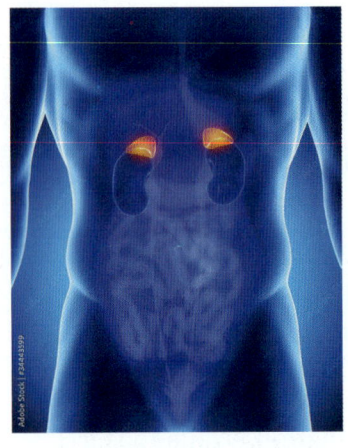

The adrenals are small organs that sit on top of the kidneys. They have a lot of blood flow, which shows their importance. Without the adrenals we would die rather quickly, because without adrenaline the effects of stress would kill us. They help us with energy, save us when we have injuries, and influence our sexual system. We often refer to them as our stress organs.

CRH (corticotropin releasing hormone) from the hypothalamus stimulates ACTH which is released by the pituitary gland. ACTH stimulates cortisol secretion by the adrenals.

Cortisol is referred to as the stress hormone. It influences carbohydrate metabolism by increasing glucose levels in the blood, increases blood pressure and decreases the immune responses. It also decreases inflammation in the body. It is catabolic hormone, meaning it is uses the energy stores and resources of the body and does not have a restorative function. Its secretion is diurnal. Therefore measuring cortisol is often most useful when done numerous times a day.

Levels that are too high or levels that are too low are not healthy.

We need to figure out how to effectively deal with stresses, in some cases stressors can be removed, but most of the time a better strategy needs to be found for "how to deal."

Make sleep a priority. Go to sleep by 10 pm every night. In this way restorative hormones can be secreted, melatonin and growth hormone. Without good sleep everything falls apart. Turn off the television by 8 pm.

Exercise is a great stress reducer. It metabolizes stress hormones, increases growth hormone levels and endorphin secretion. **Use supplements** for adrenals if needed: DHEA, Adrenal glandular, B Vitamins, and Vitamin C

The adrenals contain two main parts, the cortex or the outside, and medulla or the inside. They are a part of the endocrine system, and are important components of the HPA axis. The **HPA axis** is a term for the endocrine system that connects with the nervous system. It stands for Hypothalamus, Pituitary and Adrenal glands. The thyroid is also involved.

Adrenal stress starts with communications of the Central Nervous System (CNS) with the HPA axis: The hypothalamus releases CRH, which communicates with the Pituitary, which then releases ACTH, which stimulates the adrenals to release GC (cortisol), which in turn releases adrenaline that raises blood pressure, blood sugar, oxidants and heart rate.

Chronic stress is more about how we react to the external environment and less about what happens. It is really a choice about how we respond to what happens in our life. We often cannot change what happens to us, but we can change how we choose to react to it.

Letting go of our programmed emotional "feeling" is, at the deepest level, what we need to do. Responses based on our emotions are not what we are called to in life. Living in the Divine presence allows us as humans to respond in a divine way. If something negative or tragic has occurred to us, it can draw us closer to God, if we choose to allow it.

We need to respond in a godly way. Our feelings or emotional selves are not the problem, but rather, how we deal with those feelings. Feeling cannot be repressed or ignored. Feelings must be confronted with reason and faith. This is what makes us human and divine at the same time. This process of life calls us to reach a deeper understanding of self by allowing the spiritual self, the part connected to God, to manifest."

– Donald Yance Jr., CN, AHG

Adrenal Insufficiency Symptoms

Donald Yance Jr. describes the symptoms of deficiency as (pre-Addison's Disease condition):

- Fatigue/malaise
- Depression
- Higher risk of inflammatory conditions and autoimmune diseases
- Heart disease
- Breast cancer
- Poor concentration (ADD-like behavior)
- Inability to cope
- Imbalances in weight – under or over
- Weakness
- Dryness conditions
- Allergies
- Asthma
- Reduced libido
- Restless sleep

Adrenal Hyper-activation Symptoms

Donald Yance Jr. describes the symptoms of hyperactivity

- Anxiety
- Agitation/irritability
- Restless sleep
- Increased cholesterol
- Increased blood pressure
- Insulin resistance
- Reduced libido
- Depression
- Impaired memory/learning
- Gastrointestinal disorders
- Loss of muscle tone
- Protein loss
- Bone loss
- Skin disorders
- Reduced immune function
- Poor healing ability

> **Adrenal References**
>
> **Books**
> *Seven Symbols of Healing,*
> *12 Essential Minerals for Cellular Health*
> by David R. Card
>
> **DavesHealingNotes.com**
> Adrenal Fatigue
> Fainting

Adrenal Emotions

From ***Feelings Buried Alive Never Die*** by Karol Truman or ***Heal Your Body*** by Louise Hay:

- Feels a victim
- Feelings of being defeated
- "Don't care what happens to me" attitude
- Feelings of anxiety
- Misusing the will
- Subconscious belief that life must have burden
- Unresolved jealousies and fears
- Feeling that one must struggle for success, power or position
- Defeatism
- No longer caring for the self
- Anxiety

Adrenal Facial Diagnosis

Thin pale face

Nervous expression – stressed or anxious

Dark circle under eyes

Swollen area at the root of the nose between the eyes

Female facial hair (fine hairs)

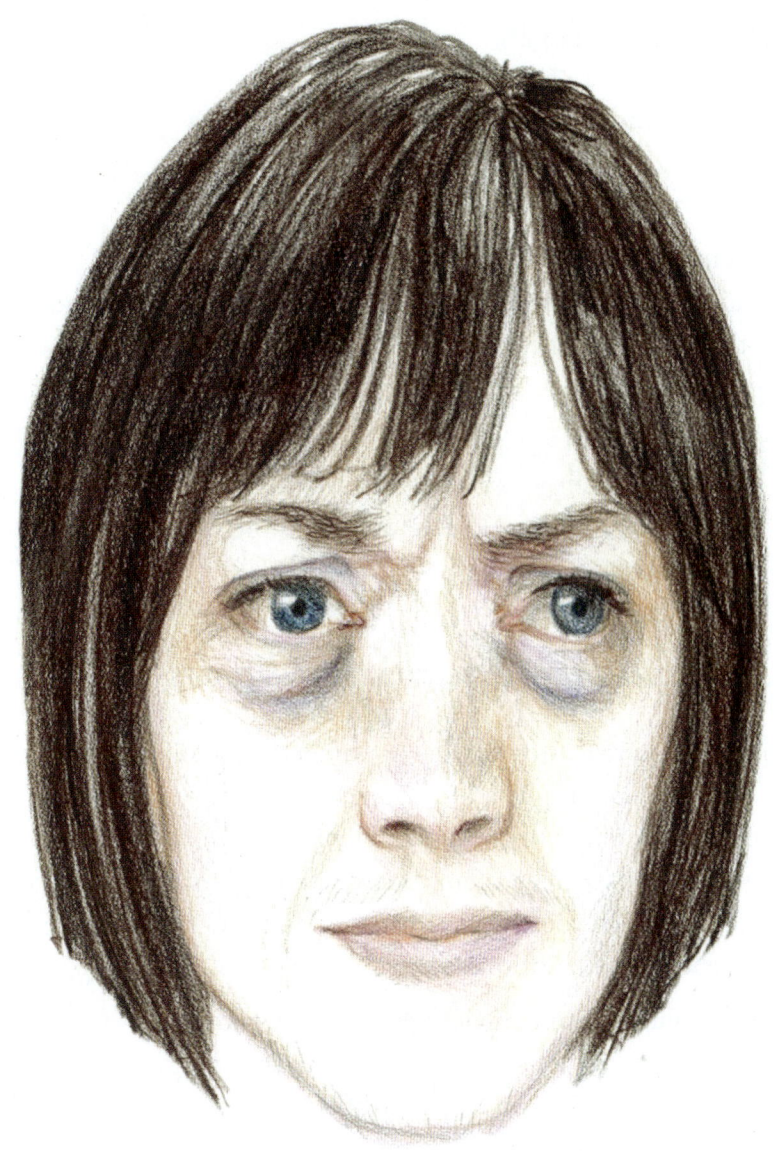

Adrenal Herbs

Ashwagandha is an adaptogen and a nervine sedative, anti-stress, memory enhancer, immune-protective.

Eleutherococcus is adaptogenic, increases endurance and concentration, used for general exhaustion and weakness.

Licorice increases the activity of cortisol and aldosterone and has pro-immune activity. It is also anti-allergy and anti-inflammatory. It can be used to help decrease use of steroid medications.

Panax ginseng or **Asian ginseng** is adaptogenic for the HPA axis, helps blood sugar control, and improves memory and learning, immune-stimulant.

Rhodiola improves depression, fatigue, and work performance; helps with chronic stress; affects the central nervous system and neurotransmitters.

Adrenal Homeopathic Medicines

Argentum nit: anticipation, apprehension and fear; periodic fatigue and weakness. Impulsive, in a hurry, craves sugar, gassy, belching. Symptoms worse with emotions; intolerant of heat, better in cool air. Performance anxiety, diarrhea from emotions.

Arsenicum album: anxiety, restlessness and exhaustion; nervous constitution, thirsty, taking sips often. Fastidious, fear of death and disease. Worse after midnight, happens periodically, aggravated upon exertion; better with heat, warm foods and drink.

Gelsemium: aching, tiredness, heaviness, weakness, soreness, dullness, apathy. Droopy eyelids, inner trembling, chills up and down back, no thirst. Worse in spring, from bad news, humidity, better in open air, bending over.

Nux vomica: collapse, fatigue, overwhelmed feeling, overactive mind, irritable, angry and impatient. Works hard and plays hard, craves spicy foods, stimulants and fats. Better from a nap, worse early in the morning and cold open air.

Phosphorus: oversensitive to ambient variables. Fatigue, dizziness after rising. Short naps help. Worse from physical or mental exertion, better with cold food and drinks.

Adrenal Cell Salts

Ferr phos: with dark circles under the eyes.

Kali phos: with nervous exhaustion.

Mag phos: with muscle cramps. Always better with heat.

The Stomach: Stomach and Stomach Ulcers

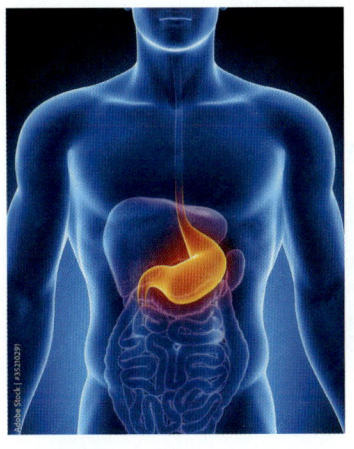

The stomach is the first mixer and separator of our nutrients, as well as creating many of the chemicals that affect the brain and thus our mental health. It needs lots of blood and circulation to produce sufficient acid to break down food. We can imagine the stomach as a caldron, and we add food to be cooked. The right amount of stomach acid is one of our first lines of defense. We must tend the fire to cook the food just right. If the "fire," our stomach acid, is too low, the food doesn't break down well, and it may not kill the viruses and bacteria that could endanger our lives. This represents low stomach acid. In our culture, there is far too much anti-acid and acid blocker usage.

The process of digestion involves the stomach, liver, gallbladder, small intestine, pancreas, and large intestine. They all play a part in good digestion which helps you avoid indigestion, gas, bloating, constipation, or diarrhea. Good digestion can help to prevent cancers, colitis and IBS, but all the above organs need to function well; it is a team effort.

Digestive problems are often hard to diagnose with modern medicine. Their treatments tend to consist of drugs that mask symptoms and cause a myriad of side effects, creating other problems. Many of these drugs are addictive. Many medications for digestive problems are acid reducing (makes you feel better in the short term), but cause long-term problems such as osteoporosis, anemia, and many immune system issues. Herbs, homeopathics and other approaches will help and often eliminate the need for drugs.

Diet: One cannot solve digestive problems without having a healthy diet. Critical items to eliminate are tobacco, alcohol, coffee, black tea, sodas, and fast foods. Next, one needs to eat fresh foods, not boxed, canned, bagged, or fast or fried foods.

Stomach Emotions

Karol Truman says, in her book ***Feelings Buried Alive Never Die***:

Stomach problems:
- Our sense of security feels threatened
- Fears new ideas
- Lack of affection
- Condemning the success of other people
- Unhappy feelings

Gastritis:
- Feeling of uncertainty
- Feelings of anxiety

Stomach Facial Diagnosis

Early thick graying hair

Small pale scar on the tip of the nose

Nose indentation (looks like a saddle)

Red nose (by itself) – chronic gastritis

White nose tip – low acid, poor digestion

Nose tip separation – gastritis, ulcer sign

Fleshy nose – ulcerative sign

Strong lines from nose to corners of the mouth

Thin male beard on the cheeks

Small upper lips – low acid

Stretched mouth opening

Vertical lines above and below the lips

Long line from the cheek to the jaw line

Pale spot in middle of lower lip –indigestion

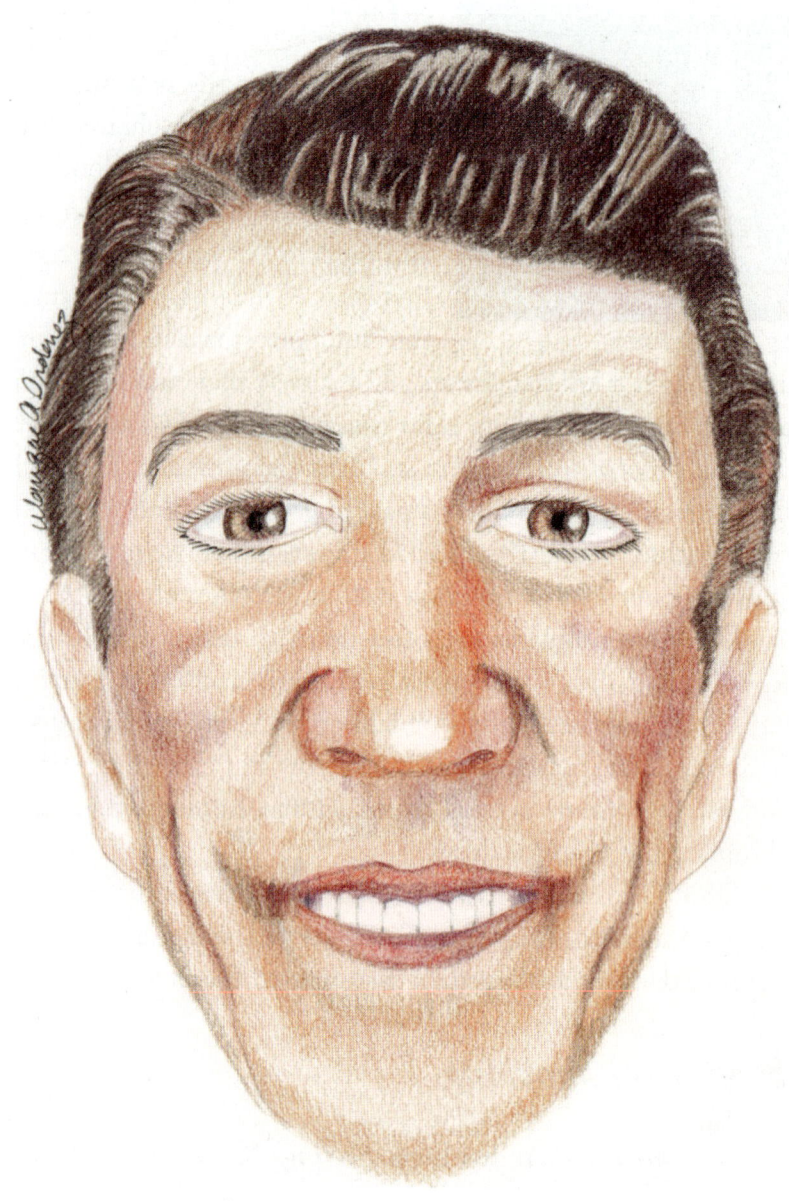

> ### Using Digestive Enzymes
>
> Using **digestive enzyme** supplements can help when a person has a severe disease process, or there is digestive debility. Immune function and digestion ability are closely related.
>
> Normal digestive function does not produce excessive gas, bloating, or indigestion. It also prevents conditions such as ulcers, irritable bowel syndrome, hemorrhoids, or diarrhea. Pancreas function is important for digestion, as it produces enzymes which aid in the digestion process. Enzymes help the body digest our food, which takes pressure off the immune system.
>
> When used on an empty stomach, the enzyme protease acts as a natural anti-inflammatory. There are other digestive enzymes as well. However, the use of herbs and homeopathics can aid the body to normalize its own enzyme production; thus, not only can we strengthen digestion, but immune function as well. If using digestive enzyme supplements, a person can start adding herbs and homeopathics until eventually achieving normal function without the need for enzymes.

Stomach Herbs

Stomach or digestive herbs can be used as teas of in capsules, usually in combination. Use them several times a day. **Bitter herbs stimulate** stomach acid and digestion.

Carminative herbs break up gas and bloating and often are high in essential oils.

Blessed thistle stimulates the liver to produce bile to digest fats and increases normal acid production.

Celery seed increases stomach acid and improves digestion.

Chamomile is one of the most important herbs to increase digestion and reduce gas and bloating while it acts as an anti-inflammatory.

Fennel breaks up gas and bloating and stimulates digestion.

Angelica stimulates stomach acid, warms a cold digestion.

Yarrow stimulates stomach acid and helps to heal leaky gut syndrome.

Fenugreek is a mild bitter, stimulating digestion and breaking up mucus.

Dandelion root stimulates stomach acid, bile production, and digestion.

Peppermint releases gas and bloating. Best if used in small amounts.

Stomach Homeopathic Medicines

Homeopathic remedies for heartburn. Pick your specific remedy by symptoms. Use in 6c or 30c potency every few minutes or as often as needed.

Remedy	Belching	Bitter taste	Bloating	Burning	Eating, after	Worse < lying down	Pressure	Sour taste	Undigested food
Antimonium Crud	✓					✓		✓	
Antimonium Tart		✓							
Argentum Nitricum	✓		✓	✓					
ARSENICUM ALBUM						✓	✓	✓	
Asafoetida	✓			✓					
Berberis		✓			✓				
Bryonia		✓							
Cactus			✓						✓
CALC CARB					✓	✓		✓	✓
Capsicum				✓			✓		
CARBO VEG				✓		✓	✓	✓	✓
Chelidonium		✓			✓				
Cinchona	✓		✓		✓				
CONIUM						✓		✓	
Graphites	✓						✓		
Iris Versicolor	✓	✓		✓		✓		✓	
Kreosotum	✓	✓							✓
LYCOPODIUM	✓		✓	✓		✓			
MAG CARB				✓			✓	✓	
NATRUM PHOS				✓	✓	✓	✓	✓	
Nux Moschata	✓			✓					
NUX VOMICA	✓	✓		✓	✓	✓	✓	✓	
Phosphorus	✓					✓	✓	✓	✓
PULSATILLA		✓		✓			✓		
Robinia		✓	✓			✓	✓	✓	
Sepia	✓	✓	✓			✓		✓	
Veratrum Album	✓			✓					

Stomach Cell Salts

Calc phos: gas, weak digestion, heartburn.

Ferr phos: sour belching, vomiting, undigested food.

Kali phos: with nervous depression, sea sickness, nausea.

Mag phos: stomach cramps, colic in babies.

Nat mur: weak stomach, heartburn, morning sickness, grief.

Nat phos: ulcers, heartburn, sour heartburn, sour vomiting.

Nat sulph: morning sickness, green vomiting.

Silicea: weak, frail, severe heartburn.

Stomach Ulcers

Stomach ulcers are common in 25- to 35-year-olds. They can develop because of a nervous condition or excess acid. Stomach cramps and vomiting may be included in symptoms. Pain is frequently from one-half to two hours after eating. Pain can radiate to the back or chest areas. Nights can be bad as the stomach is empty and the acid can be irritating. Ulcers can be consequence of poor diet, or happen at onset of menses in proportion to fat in the diet.

Stomach Ulcer Facial Diagnosis

Early graying of hair

Sparse facial hair in men

Pale nose

Deep lines above lips

Deep lines from nostrils to corners of mouth

Small lips

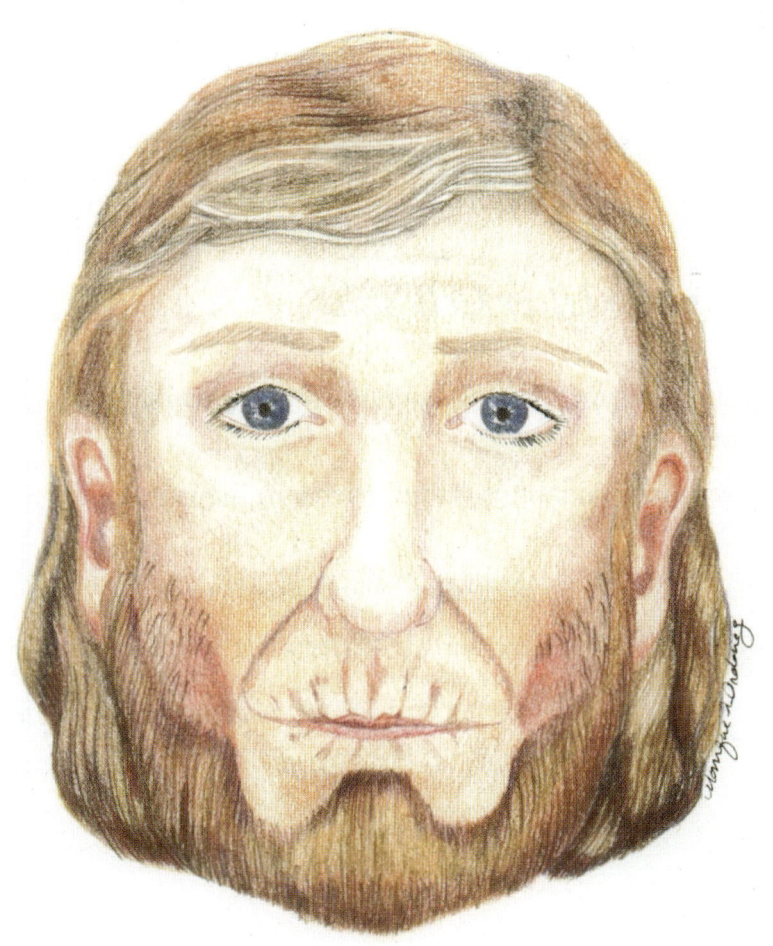

Stomach Ulcer Homeopathic Medicine

Anacardium: ulcer worse on empty stomach, relieved by eating food (painful hunger). Hypoglycemia, anger, insulting, critical, absent-minded, spacey; nervous eating to relieve symptoms.

Argentum nit: gnawing pain in stomach, sharp pains radiating outward; made worse by breathing deeply. Violent retching, green diarrhea, gas, bloating, intense craving for chocolate. Binging on sweets, which aggravate symptoms.

Arsenicum album: burning like fire, made better with hot drinks. Blood in stools. If ulcer perforated or food poisoning present: ejecting from both ends.

Bismuth: indigestion, vomiting of cold drinks, vomiting 15 minutes after ingestion. Burning pain relieved bending backwards or forwards. Restlessness worse immediately after cold drinks.

Kali bichromicum: pain in small spots worse after eating; heaviness and swelling after eating, worsened by beer; can alternate with diarrhea plus arthritis in various joints throughout body. More frequent with heavy, glutinous people.

Lycopodium: right-sided pains, worse 4-8 pm; belching, bloating, burning, worse lying down.

Mercurius corrosive: blood in stool; use if normal Mercury is not going deep enough.

Nux vomica: stimulates hydrochloric acid production. Blood in stool. History of bad diet; worse when upset or angry (yelling and screaming), also when suppressing anger. Better with warm drinks, worsened with spicy foods.

Uranium nit: diabetes; piercing pain from ulcers in pyloric area. Epigastric pain, emaciation, weakness, anemia, coffee-ground vomit (mostly in cancer).

Stomach Ulcer Cell Salts

Kali phos: empty stomach, must eat often, nausea, motion sick.

Nat mur: weakness, isolation, grief, burning stomach pains.

Nat phos: peptic ulcer, sour belching and vomiting.

Nat sulph: with heartburn, gas, green bile sour vomit.

Silicea: shy, delicate, stomach gnawing pain, burning in pit of stomach.

Stomach References

Books

Seven Symbols of Healing, 12 Essential Minerals for Cellular Health by David R. Card

DavesHealingNotes.com
Canker sores
Food poisoning
Gastroparesis
Heartburn
Indigestion
Parasite cleans
Stomach ulcers

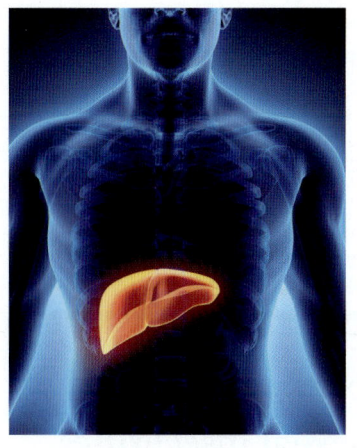

The Liver

The liver is one of our most important organs, as it has six-to-eight hundred different functions, many not yet discovered. Its main function is to **detoxify** chemicals produced by living (metabolic wastes), and from pollution and other toxins such as medications.

It has 3 main detoxification processes. Phase 1 is water soluble foods or chemical compounds; phase 2 is fat soluble foods or chemical compounds: phase 3 includes the Kupffer cells that act as part of the immune system to destroy invasive bacteria and viruses. See **Liver Function Herbs** below.

We need only to know how to recognize the liver signs and the tools to keep it healthy.

Signs of liver problems:

- Discomfort in the right side of the lower rib area
- Any right-sided disturbance
- A visible hump below ribs on the right side
- Bloated abdomen full of water
- Blue veins on the abdomen (portal vein stasis)
- Brown beer-looking urine
- Clay or white-colored stools
- Flat, white opaque fingernails or chronic white spots in nails
- Skin thickening on palms of hand
- Change in female genital hair growth
- Thinning or loss of male chest hair
- Enlarged breasts on men with very little chest hair
- Chronic redness on palms of hands, or redness of the thumbs and small finger bases.
- Headaches, often on right forehead and temples
- Hemorrhoids
- Open sores in the throat
- Red varnished appearance of tongue
- Yellowish to brownish coating on tongue
- Right leg can't extend as far as the left
- Skin cool and clammy
- Yellowish to brownish appearance of gums
- Low sex drive and thin skin
- Yellow and itching skin

Liver weakening foods, substances, emotions: coffee (regular or decaf), black tea, alcohol, recreational drugs, prescription drugs, many over-the-counter drugs, antibiotics, anti-depressants, animal products including eggs; anger.

Liver strengthening foods: beets, range-fed or organic beef, red-colored foods, and foods naturally rich in iron such as dark leafy green vegetables.

Liver Emotions

Anonymous Author

Negative:	**Positive:**
Anger	Responsible
Disappointment	Transformation
Hostile	Happiness
Shameful	Content
Envy	Conscientious
Spiteful	Reliable
Irritable	Firm
Abusive	Careful
Resentful	Grateful
Rage	Pleased

Kurt Tepperwein says, "Self doubt or sexual insecurities, and depression, are signs of a diseased liver.

Also when one wants to take on new ideas, the liver regulates the release of old ones.

A healthy liver helps the body get rid of false ideas."

Liver Facial Diagnosis

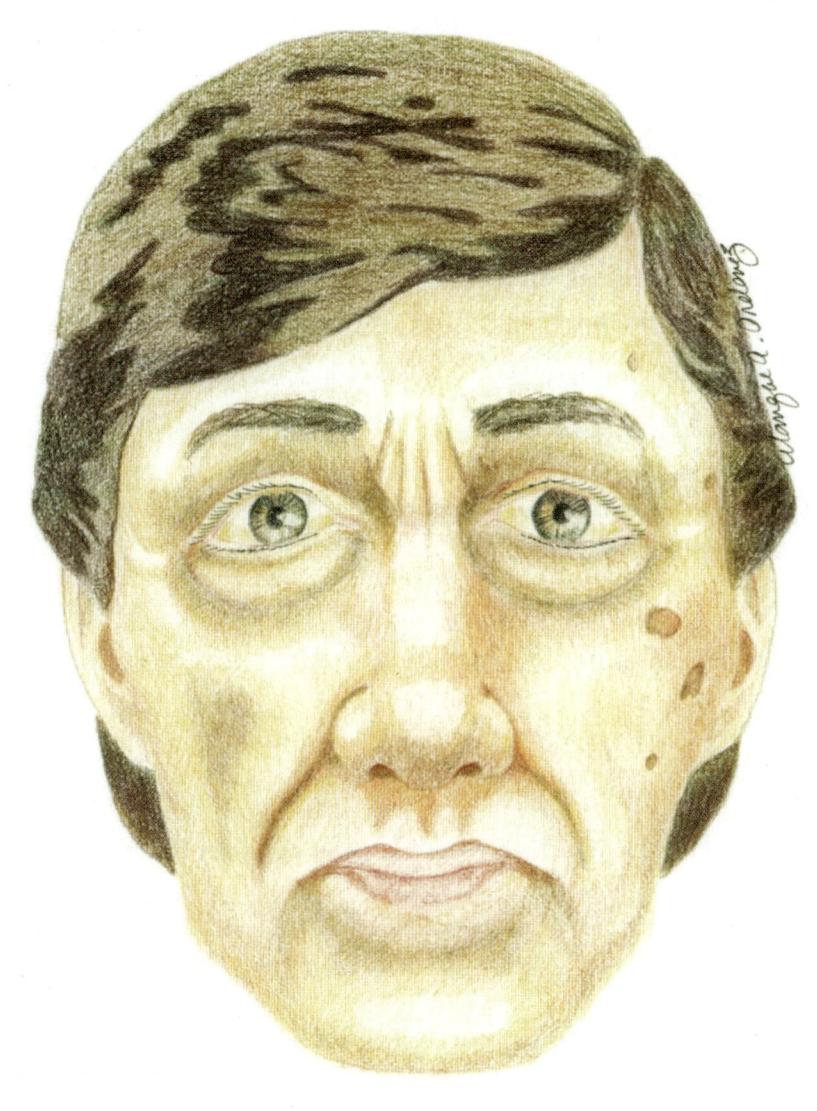

Yellow skin coloring

Horizontal and diagonal lines on the forehead

Brown spots on the borders of the hair

Ears, knot at the base of the right ear attachment

Vertical line between the eyebrows

Eye region, cholesterol deposits that look like yellow pimples

Eyelids, lower lid swelling with spider veins

Brown around the eyes

Brown or yellow pigmentation of the sclera of the eye

Nose, copper-colored dark points

Saddle of the nose thickened

Spider veins on the wings of the nose

Strong right-sided nasal labial line

Cheek, sagging right cheek

Cheeks, sunken with a slight yellow appearance

Pale lips

Lips, thickening of the lower lip as well as under the lips

Acne or pimples around the mouth

Wrinkles at the corner of the mouth

Jowl skin area translucent

Neck becomes thin

Other signs: Nosebleeds

Liver Function Herbs

As noted above, Phase 1 is water soluble foods or chemical compounds, phase 2 is fat soluble foods or chemical compounds, and phase 3 includes the Kupffer cells that act like part of the immune system. Use more than one herb; several herbs work better to improve all three liver functions

Phase I detoxification where toxins are water soluble:

Grape seed extract

Green tea (and phase II)

Milk Thistle (and phase II)

St. John's wort

Turmeric (and phase II)

Phase II detoxification where toxins are fat soluble toxins:

Cruciferous vegetables

Garlic

Horse radish root

Mustard seed

Rosemary

Sage

Schizandra (and phase I)

Turmeric (and phase I)

Watercress leaf

Phase III detoxification where Kupfer cells act like the immune system:

Echinacea

Andropraphis

Cat's Claw

Astragalus

Bio-transformation support using blood-cleansing herbs to strengthen the liver:

Burdock root

Figwort

Red clover

Yellow dock

Liver Herbs

Bitter herbs and those that increase bile to remove toxins are called cholagogues. Adaptogen herbs help improve energy or help with stress relief. Some are tonic which improve liver function.

Apple is a liver tonic, helps to improve liver function.

Artichoke is a bitter, liver/gallbladder support (helping lower cholesterol and triglycerides); helps pancreas to release digestive enzymes.

Blessed thistle is a liver tonic.

Cascara sagrada is a liver tonic, good for constipation.

Dandelion is a general liver tonic and cleanser.

Fennel breaks up gas.

Horehound is a bitter herb great for the liver, as well as being known for upper respiratory health.

Licorice supports healthy stomach mucosal lining and digestive function.

Milk thistle is tonic and liver protector.

Red Root works with the liver as well as the spleen.

Rosehips aids in digestion (helping the liver to release bile), and is rich in Vitamin C and bioflavonoids.

Turmeric in Ayurvedic practices has been used for liver-gallbladder, as well as joint function.

Wild yam releases gas, protects the liver.

Wormwood is a liver tonic, digestive and kills worms.

Liver Homeopathic Medicines

Arsenicum album: burning pains, restlessness. Liver and spleen enlarged and painful; hepatitis from food poisoning.

Belladonna: inflammation and right-sided; red, hot, sudden and throbbing.

Berberis vulgaris: radiating, sharp pains.

Bryonia: mainly right-sided stabbing pains, everything is worse with movement. Feels better lying on right side.

Chelidonuium: pain under right shoulder blade.

Cinchona: bloating. Problems after excessive fluid loss.

Iodum: feels hot, has ravenous appetite.

Magnesia mur: jaundice. Liver enlarged; bloated abdomen with yellow coated tongue. Inability to lie on the liver area.

Mercurius sol: excess saliva, temperature sensitive, bad breath, liver enlarged and hard. Low bile output. Exhaustion.

Natrum sulph: hepatitis; sore, tender, painful liver. Worsens from damp cold weather.

Nux vomica: toxic liver from drugs, chemicals, and alcohol. Food sits in stomach like a stone.

Phosphorus: burning pains, congested liver, acute hepatitis, fatty liver.

Podophyllum: diarrhea, jaundice. Sore and painful. Better with rubbing.

Sepia: estrogen dominance; low sex drive, irritable. Liver pains on movement. Liver sore and painful, relieved by lying on right side. Aching, throbbing, shooting pains in liver area.

Liver Cell Salts

To create a cell salt solution, use an 8 - 32 ounce water bottle, put in cell salts that apply to you and shake to dissolve tablets, then sip on this formula all day. For maximum results use for 6 to 8 months.

Kali mur is used to get rid of mucus and reduce inflammation of the liver.

Kali sulph is specific for excess bodily pigmentation on the skin (sometimes seen as liver spots and other colorations). There is also a yellow to brown skin tone from bile salts that have difficulty being expelled from the body.

Nat sulph for excess alcohol consumption (or excessive use of sugars), eventually showing up as a red nose.

Mag phos shows up as "magnesium red" on the face and helps to reduce liver and gallbladder cramping.

Liver References

Books

Homeopathy for Today, Facial Diagnosis of Cell Salt Deficiency, 12 Essential Minerals for Cellular Health, Seven Symbols of Healing by David R. Card

DavesHealingNotes.com
Liver Cleanse
Cholesterol

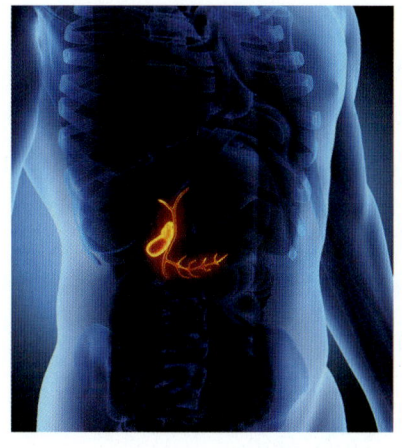

The Gallbladder

The gallbladder is a sack that sits beneath the center of the liver, located under the ribs on the right side of the abdomen. Its size is approximately 8 cm long and 4 cm wide, and consists of three walls: the first allows it to expand: the second is for contraction, and the third is connective tissue.

Many consider an imbalance in the gallbladder to be anger or bitterness. The Bible talks about people being in the "gall of bitterness." There appears to be a connection to the function of the ego. Too much or too little causes imbalance. One of our common sayings in America is that a person "has a lot of gall"; while in China they say a person has "a big gallbladder."

This organ stores and concentrates bile. The liver produces 600-800 ml of unconcentrated bile, to be stored and concentrated in the gallbladder, which holds 20 to 50 ml of concentrated bile, ready for use when fatty foods enter the duodenum as a result of cholecystokinin release. Bile serves several functions:

- To emulsify fat, breaking it down, to be utilized by the body in the form of micelles
- Lubrication for more efficient bowel movements
- Binds up toxins to be released in the bowel movement

Gallbladder Problems

Two main problems of the gallbladder are **inflammation (cholecystitis)** and **gallstones (cholelithiasis)**. These two problems account for almost twenty percent of short term hospital stays. In the United States nearly half a million gallbladders are removed, and may affect as many as 20 million people.

Gallbladder inflammation is almost always associated with gallstones and distention (gas) and often a bacterial infection.

Gallstones are composed mainly of cholesterol (yellow-greenish) or bilirubin (pigment stones). If smaller than 8mm they can pass on their own, which causes indigestion and other digestive upsets. Larger stones can obstruct the bile duct. This develops as sudden pain and sometimes climaxes in 30 to 60 minutes; other times pain will last 2 to 8 hours. According to authorities, many gallstones are caused by medical drugs that affect the liver.

Causes of gallbladder problems arise from a diet too rich in fats or the heavy standard American diet (SAD), and also from consuming too many toxins. Western medicine offers to cut out your gallbladder, nearly the only solution it has; but be careful because gallbladder surgery leaves the system in a random flow of unconcentrated bile from liver into the intestine. This often results in gas, bloating and indigestion. Changing to a healthy diet is one of the only ways to eliminate the continued influx of toxins and poisons.

In Reflexology terms, the **gallbladder reflex areas** include the tip of the right shoulder blade, as well as the right upper shoulder area. Another area is just below, and to the left of, the right nipple.

Gallbladder Emotions

Anonymous Author

Negative:	Positive:
Bitterness	Positive
Obstinate	Motivated
Dejection	Options
Rage	Forgiving
Self-righteous	Assertive
Bored	Jovial
Passive	Devoted
Helpless	Honest
Feeling inadequate	Courage

The Chinese saw the emotions of the gallbladder: "Sour nature, such as sour temper, hypochondria, lack of calm, irritability, fears, anxieties, and in short, all that is bitter, sharp, tart, biting, etc…"

– from *Chinese system of Healing*, pgs. 53-54

Gallbladder Facial Diagnosis

Dark hair, especially in women, is a predisposition to gallbladder/liver diseases

Eyebrows, raised right eyebrow

Eyes, yellow

Eyes, right eye pupil enlarged

Eyes, yellow sclera-jaundice

Cheeks, pale yellow coloring

Red face

Nose, red with dark points (dots)

Nose, nasolabial line is deeper on right side – painful gallbladder

Mouth, yellowish coloring

Mouth corner wrinkles

Teeth yellow

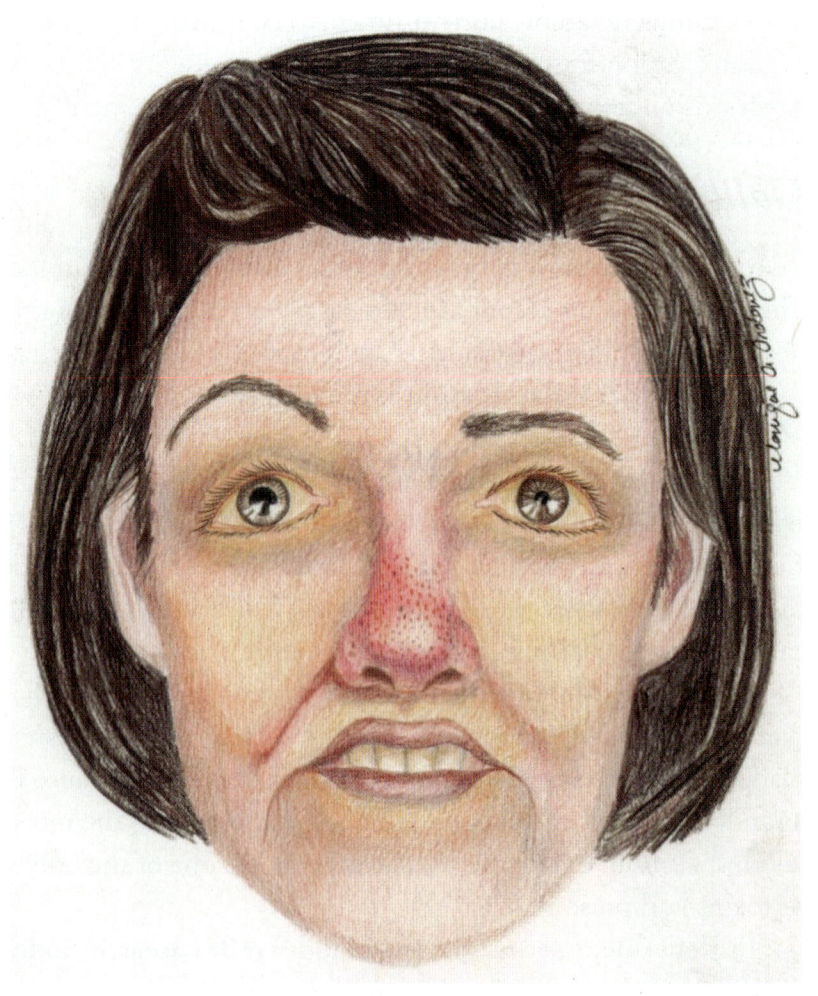

Gallbladder Herbs

Most of the herbs for gallbladder are cholagogues, that is, they stimulate the liver to produce more bile. Bile has several different functions as discussed above, so these herbs help to prevent or eliminate gallstones and help the liver to function properly as well. They are all bitter as well, which supports healthy liver function.

Artichoke, along with most liver remedies, is useful in helping the liver to produce more bile.

Burdock root is a mild cholagogue as well as helping the colon detox

Dandelion root works well with Oregon grape root and benefits the liver.

Goldenseal also helps the mucus membranes and acts like an antibiotic. (Expensive and scarce)

Gravel root as dissolvent, use with Marshmallow.

Hydrangea is a dissolvent and "cuts" sharp edges off stones.

Gentian is a cholagogue that improves digestion as well.

Hops is a bitter tonic that also affects hormones, pain and sleep.

Lemon juice is a mild cholagogue.

Marshmallow helps soothe the tissues when stones break up so they won't hurt so much.

Motherwort is a cholagogue that also works on thyroid, hormones, heart palpitations, and digestion.

Oregon grape root is a great cholagogue that also contains berberine, a component that works like an antibiotic.

Gallbladder References

Books

Homeopathy for Today,
12 Essential Minerals for
Cellular Health
by David R. Card

DavesHealingNotes.com
Gallstones
Heartburn

Gallbladder Homeopathic Medicines

Gallbladder pain with bilious temperament, melancholic person, infection, blocked duct, severe pain in bile duct (info from Dr. Robin Murphy).

Berberis: gallstones, colic, sciatica, back, nerve problems. Radiating pain to back, sides, abdomen; sticking pain (stays there). Symptoms come and go quickly, worse motion, worse pressure. Breathing difficult, shallow. Clay-colored stools, jaundice. Compare to Bryonia.

Bryonia: worsens with motion, better pressure, better lying on painful side. Dry mouth, thirst for cold water.

Carduus mar: sticking in gallbladder area, tearing with cramps, and spasms. Worsened with pressure and touching liver area, better lying on left side. Intense nausea, bilious vomiting (dark green, acid bitter taste). For liver use Carduus, Chel, and Tarax.

Chelidonium: sticking cramps and spasms in gallbladder, pain beneath right scapula. Yellow tongue, jaundice; desire for warm drinks, worse 4-8 pm, better eating and drinking.

China (Cinchona): hypersensitive to touch; better with deep pressure, worsened by jarring. Abdomen distended, gas, bloating, must loosen clothing. NWS (Never well since) gallbladder surgery, not better passing gas.

Dioscorea: gallstone attacks, wants to stretch backwards, chest pains, cutting pains, worse evening.

Lycopodium: worse 4 to 8 pm with indigestion, mostly right-sided pains. Worsened by lying on right side. Compare to China, Chel.

Natrum sulph: liver/gallbladder remedy. Jaundice, worse 4-5 a.m. Made better lying on right side.

Gallbladder inflammation, recommendations from Dr. Gawlik: **Bryonia, Chelidonium, Taraxicum, Pyrogenium, Hedra Helix**

Gallstones (cholecystopathy) with high fever, colic pains, and circulatory problems: **Belladonna, Berberis, Colocynthis, Dioscorea, Mandragora, Carduus mar, Taraxacum, Bryonia, Chelidonium.**

Gallbladder Cell Salts

Calc phos: indigestion, acid.

Calc fluor: connective tissue.

Kali sulph: supports liver (bile).

Mag phos: gallstone colic, spasms.

Nat sulph: gallbladder disorders. Clawing pain in gallbladder area. Stimulates liver to produce more bile to clean the gallbladder.

The Pancreas: Blood Sugar and Type II Diabetes

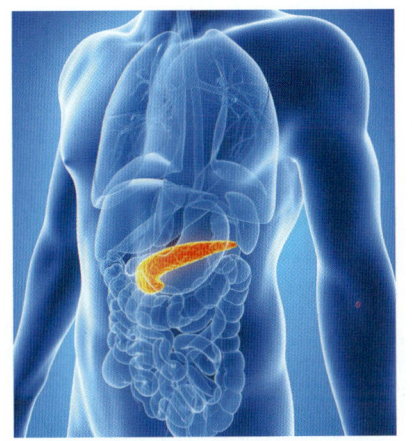

The pancreas is a glandular organ that sits behind the stomach and serves two functions:
1. Endocrine function of **excreting insulin** to help sugars be used by the cells for energy. Diabetes is an excess of sugar in the blood when the pancreas can't produce insulin or when the cells become insulin resistant.
2. An exocrine function when the pancreas releases **digestive enzymes and sodium bicarb** to facilitate breakdown of foods and absorption in the small intestine.

Aside from diabetes, pancreas imbalance can cause hypoglycemia and indigestion, which can result in inflammation and more.

Pancreas Emotions
Anonymous Author

Negative:	Positive:
Judgmental	Accepting
Disappointed	Satisfied
Sadness	Happiness
Shock	Comforted
Wanting control	Letting go
Ashamed of your past	Forgiving
Joy of living is gone	Joyful

"To taste the sweetness of life, you must have the power to forget the past."

– Nishan Panwar

Pancreas and Blood Sugar Regulation

Blood sugar regulation starts with the pancreas, but is connected to the adrenal glands. The adrenals' function is to release a chemical messenger that converts glycogen in the liver to glucose and increase blood sugars. The insulin is released from pancreas, and its job is to reduce blood sugar by permitting sugar into the body's cells to be used as fuel.

Whenever one of these systems is not functioning properly the blood sugars are imbalanced and one feels poorly. **High blood sugar** can produce a dull feeling over the short term and other more serious complications over the long term. **Low blood sugar** affects the memory, thinking, and may cause dizziness. Blood sugar normalization may require several hours or longer to regulate.

One author recommends an apricot and pineapple diet to cleanse the pancreas while another author recommends Marshmallow, Astragalus and Spirulina to calm the pancreas.

Blood Sugar Facial Diagnosis

Broken blood vessels on the face – metabolism disturbance

Eyebrows, thick hair growth between the eyes

Eyes, brown pigmentation in the iris

Nose, skin thickening of lines from the outer nose to corner of mouth

Cheeks red

Mouth, small or thin upper lip – also sign of low stomach acid

Breath fruity

Mouth, thickening of the tissue next to the corners

Tongue, cracked vertically down the center and short horizontal

Other body signs

Rapid weight loss

Claylike skin spots below the ribs

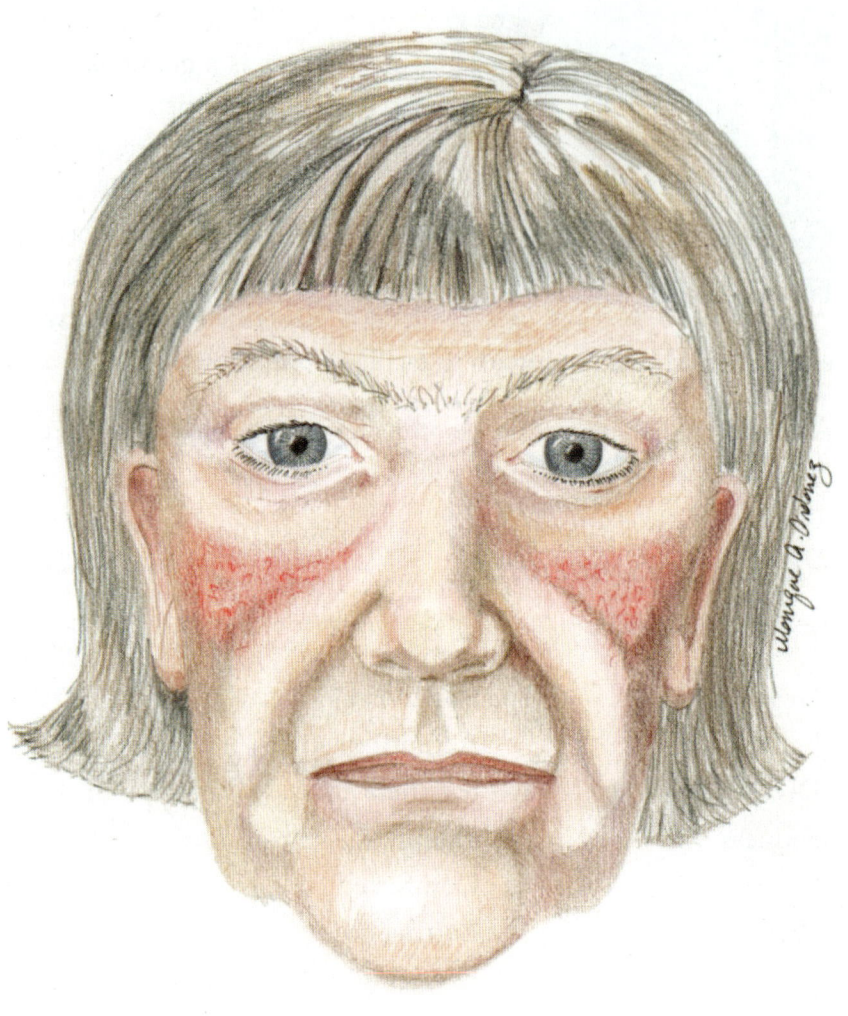

Pancreas Herbs

Aloe vera may lower blood sugar levels in type 1 diabetes.

Blue Flag (10 drops 3 times a day) to support healthy pancreas function.

Eleutherococcus may lower elevated blood sugar.

Mistletoe stimulates the release of insulin from the beta cells (insulin-producing) in the pancreas.

Fenugreek seeds may lower elevated blood sugar levels, improve glucose tolerance, and reduce urinary excretion of glucose in type 1 diabetics.

Flax seed meal helps reduce sugar metabolism.

Green tea may lower blood sugar; may also regenerate inactive beta cells.

Holy basil helps to absorb insulin more efficiently and help a person to lower the dose of insulin medications.

Gymnema sylvestre helps normalize blood sugar levels.

Yarrow may help to regenerate the pancreas.

Pancreas Homeopathic Medicine

Acute pancreas disease and endocrine pancreatic tumors are not effectively treated with homeopathy alone. Homeopathy is to be used with other measures. Pancreatic symptoms are very changeable and remedies are often hard to distinguish.

Carbo veg: venous congestion with fading pancreatitis, circulation disturbances. Body pale, cyanotic; nausea, loud gas; wants cool air, better with cold, movement, worsened with rest, warmth, fatty foods. Low tolerance for milk.

Chionanthus virg: pancreatitis, reduced appetite, bitter tasting heartburn. Stools dark, stinking; urine also stinks. Made better with rest, lying, eating; worse from cold and movement.

Chinchona: acute or chronic pancreatitis. Full feeling, bloating, vomiting without relief, bitter taste in mouth. Desires for sweets; worsened with legumes and milk.

Hypoglycemia Homeopathic Medicines

Notes from Dr. Robin Murphy N.D.

#1 Phosphoru: spicy, weak, craves cold drinks.

Nat mur: grief, dry, craves salty foods, feels isolated.

Argentum nit: left sided gas bloating, flatulence, panic attacks, anxiety, nervousness, most severe hypoglycemia, eats a whole box of chocolates, fear of the future.

Pancreas Cell Salts

Kali mur: mucus cleanser.

Kali sulph: main pancreas strengthener.

Mag phos: muscle utilization.

Nat mur: dryness all over, salt cravings.

Nat sulph: water regulation, liver involvement.

Pancreas References

Books

Facial Diagnosis of Cell Salt Deficiencies, 12 Essential Minerals for Cellular Health by David R. Card

DavesHealingNotes.com
Diabetes Type II
Diabetes, neuropathy
Low Carb Diet
Peripheral Neuropathy

Pancreas and Type II Diabetes

Diabetes is a complex disease that creates an overload of sugars which must be eliminated by the kidneys. Type II Diabetes can be the result of subconscious choices, living an unbalanced lifestyle, and unhelpful personal belief systems.

This metabolic toxic overload of sugars can create conditions or diseases such as heart disease, stroke, high blood pressure, blindness, kidney disease, nervous system damage, need for amputations, periodontal disease, depression, and even several autoimmune disorders.

These problems may be caused by, or made worse by conventional medicines (drugs). Drugs only suppress the body and control blood sugar levels. While this can be lifesaving, it doesn't address the underlying conditions. Drugs may also be a crutch for not changing diet or lifestyle, as many diabetics often eat anything they want, counting on drugs to compensate for poor diet.

Adult-onset diabetes (Type II) is the result of a **weak pancreas and endocrine function**. It is also related to digestion, stress, liver function, and more. Many diabetics have a poor diet, lack of exercise, and experience severe stress.

Cells throughout the body become toxic and cannot utilize sugar, even though there may be an abundance of insulin. Changing diet, lifestyle, exercising, and getting to a healthy weight can change one who has diabetes into a health person.

Artificial sweeteners are chemicals that must be deactivated by the liver which expends great energy to detoxify the body. They cheat the body, even though they taste sweet, triggering the pancreas into releasing insulin into the blood. A better strategy is to consume more fiber-rich foods in order to slow the release of sugar into the system. This allows the pancreas to adapt to sugars that fuel the body.

Nutrition for Diabetes

Cod liver oil counteracts neuropathy in diabetics.

Fish oil lowers blood sugar levels.

Chromium improves insulin sensitivity.

Vanadium increases glucose uptake in diabetics.

Berberine extract (herbal) helps to regulate blood sugar in diabetics.

Pancreas: Type II Diabetes Facial Diagnosis

Gray hair in young people

Dull hair

Eyes, spider veins specifically on the outer corners

Red cheeks

Corners of the mouth thickening

Nose line thickening near the nasolabial line

Upper lip smaller

Lower lip drooping

Under lower lip a sharp blue line

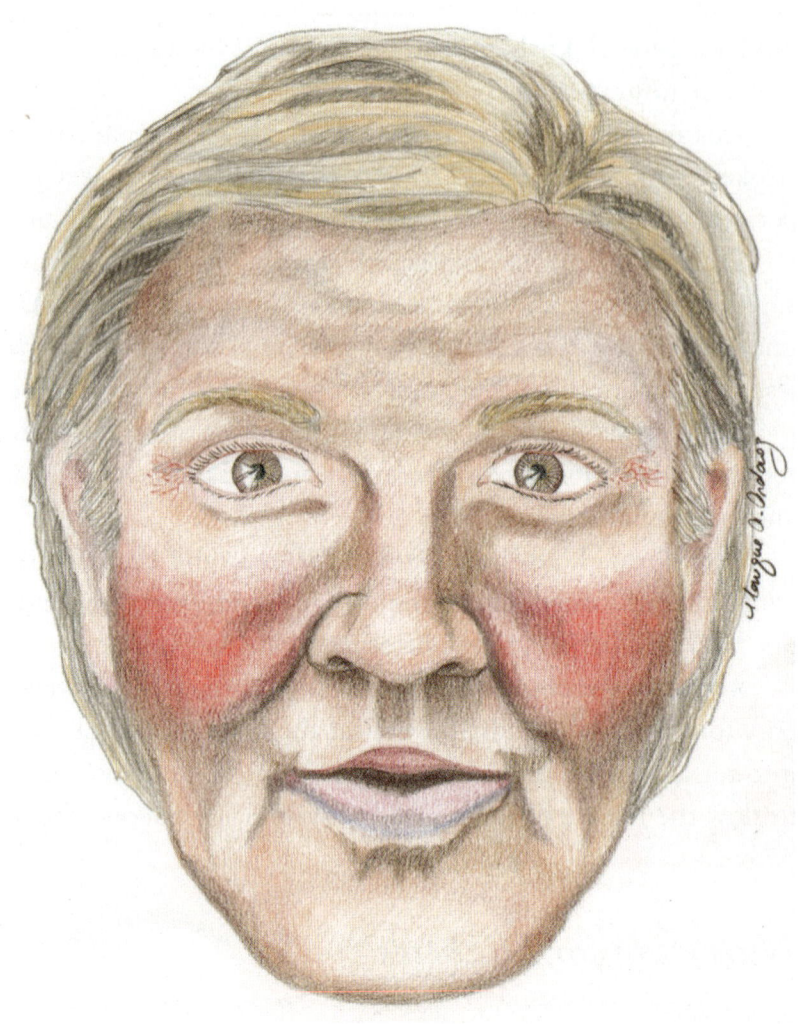

Pancreas: Type II Herbs Diabetes

Diabetes herbs can be used in a combination to support adrenals (stress raises blood sugar), remove mucus, improve digestion and protect the urinary system.

Cinnamon bark is a spice used around the world; helpful in maintaining healthy glucose levels and improves digestion.

Elecampane is decongestant, helps maintain healthy pancreas function.

Eleutherococcus helps maintain the endocrine system, including the adrenals. It is an adaptogen to help the body adapt to stress; greater stress equals higher blood sugar, lower stress equals lower blood sugar.

Oregon grape root supports liver function and improves bile for better digestion and fat metabolism.

Saw palmetto helps maintain healthy blood sugar levels by regulating the urinary system.

Spirulina is a good protein source, high in minerals and supports healthy pancreas function.

Uva ursi is helpful to the pancreas because it assists the kidneys in releasing sugars.

> **Physical & Dietary Rules for Healthy Blood Sugar**
>
> Avoid refined or simple sugars
>
> Avoid artificial sweeteners
>
> Avoid animal fats and trans fats
>
> Support pancreas with herbs, homeopathics
>
> Check your emotions; work on releasing with flower essences or homeopathics
>
> Exercise – increases cells' sensitivity to insulin

Pancreas: Type II Diabetes Homeopathic Medicines

Acetic acid: anemia, prostration, debility (emaciation), oily greasy skin, ill-effects of anesthesia, diabetic edema, overweight.

Bovista: diabetes with circulatory problems, bleeding, stuttering, clumsy.

Bryonia: thirst, dryness with headaches (Nat mur and Bry).

Calcarea carb: middle-age overweight, stocky, desires sweets, salt, eggs. Elderly cramps in legs and calves in bed, poor circulation, diabetes with obesity.

Helonias (similar to lactic acid and phosphoric acid): extreme exhaustion, fatigue, emaciation and debility. Depressed gloomy personality. Restless, problems with uterus and ovaries. Long labor and exhaustion.

Pancreas: Type II Diabetes Homeopathic Medicines continued…

Lactic acid: exhaustion, history of overwork, collapse. Muscle aches, sensitive skin, liver problems associated with extreme thirst; nausea, voracious appetite, dryness of skin and mouth. Lactic acid from overexertion. Use Calc carb also, 3 times a day for joint aches.

Lycopodium: liver and digestive problems. Worse 4 - 8 pm, gas and bloating, low self-esteem.

Phosphoric acid: diabetes with one who desires soda pop. Exhaustion, emotional flatness from grief or loss.

Phosphorus: diabetes with overstimulation, causing exhaustion. Afraid of the dark and thunderstorms; open and friendly person.

Plumbum met: diabetes with slow progression, including nerve damage which affects walking and muscular coordination.

Syzygium: this is helpful used in low potency (6X), 2 pellets 3 times a day, as a transition remedy to change to a healthier diet.

Tarantula hispida: diabetes with nerve damage, hyperactive behaviors.

Terebinthina: diabetes with kidney damage from excess sugar.

Uranium nitricum: diabetes with emaciation, abdominal swelling, and swelling of all tissues.

Pancreas: Diabetes Cell Salts

Calc phos: with irritability, wants to travel, hard to please.

Ferr phos: with anemia, nosebleeds.

Kali phos: with nervous disorders, brain fog, overwhelming stress.

Mag phos: with muscle and neurological disorders.

Nat mur: with dryness, grief, herpes.

Nat sulph: associated with head injury, or person worse from damp conditions.

Silicea: with frailty, shyness, frequent urination, sweating.

Pancreas: Type II Diabetes References

Books

Facial Diagnosis of Cell Salt Deficiencies, 12 Essential Minerals for Cellular Health by David R. Card

DavesHealingNotes.com
Diabetes Type II
Diabetes, neuropathy
Low Carb Diet
Peripheral Neuropathy

The Colon: Large Intestine

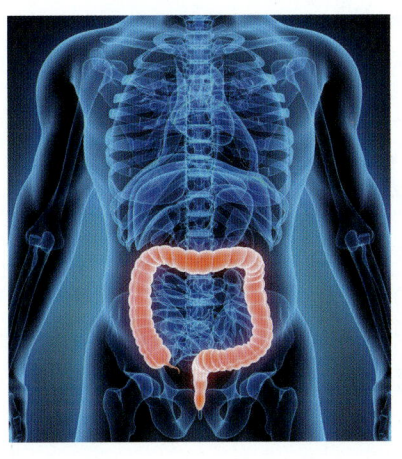

Colon health starts with chewing our food well which releases saliva that contains enzymes to start the digestive process. The stomach contains large amounts of hydrochloric acid that breaks up the food into chime. Next, the chime goes into the small intestine past the pancreas and gallbladder. The pancreas ideally neutralizes the stomach acid and inserts a copious amount of enzymes. The gallbladder then puts out bile to break down fats, sends toxins into the colon for release, and lubricates the bowels to keep them moving. These upper parts must work right for good colon health.

The small intestine is wrapped in muscles to create peristalsis and keep things moving. With a surface area the size of a football field, most of the nutrient absorption occurs here. There are also large amounts of probiotics that help the digestion process when it works right.

Next, the food goes to the large intestine (colon) where the last of the minerals are extracted. The large intestine is over 6 feet long in adults. What remains, after the colon, enters the rectum and is released into the toilet as feces.

Eating for Colon health

Eat slowly and with joy. Fresh fruits and vegetables contain lots of fiber as well as enzymes which help you avoid constipation. They also feed the probiotics in your gut.

The colon needs prebiotics (which help with digestion). If you have recently used an antibiotic, you may need 10 billion a day for one to three months.

Colon health requires a diet free of tobacco, alcohol, soda, fast foods, and excessive coffee.

Colon Emotions

From ***Feelings Buried Alive Never Die*** by Karol Truman or ***Heal Your Body*** by Louise Hay:

Colon: bottled up hate

Colon Inflammation (Colitis:
- Overly concerned with order (lose freedom)
- Excessive worry
- Feelings of oppression
- Feelings of defeat
- Feeling a need for more affection

Constipation:
- Constantly fretting
- Unwilling or release old feelings and beliefs
- Resisting the flow of life
- Feelings of anxiety
- Unresolvable problems – determined to carry on

Diarrhea:
- Rejecting the visualization of something you don't want to accept
- Wanting to be done with someone or something
- Running away from a situation
- Fear of something in the present
- Obsessed with order

Colon References

Books

Homeopathy for Today, Facial Diagnosis of Cell Salt Deficiencies, by David R. Card

DavesHealingNotes.com

Acid reflux
Anemia
Celiac disease
Cholera
Colic, babies
Colitis, ulcerative
Constipation
Colon cleanse
Crohn's disease
Diverticulitis
Gastro-paresis
Heartburn
Hemorrhoids
IBS (irritable bowel)
Leaky gut syndrome
Stomach, indigestion
Stomach, ulcers

Colon Facial Diagnosis

(Women are more likely to have colon problems than men.)

Hair brittle

Brown liver spots on forehead and facial pigmentation

Ear areas brown

Bluish eye area in children – parasites

Hollow eyes

Lower eye sacks, very wide

Red face

Line from middle of chin area to where naso-labial line follows

Brown mouth area

Corners of mouth, polished pale red

Strong horizontal line under the mouth

Liver spots on the hands

Long vertical lines on the fingernails

Lips: upper lip=small intestine, lower lip=large intestine

Lower lip thicker than normal – large intestine enlargement

Bad breath

Tongue, vertical stripes that consist of white foam – colon fermentation

Tongue, coated, cracked, with red spots on the tip – colon spasms

Tongue, dry with a red stripe down the center – colon inflammation with diarrhea and bloating

Tongue, feels dry but looks damp – colon deficiency

Fingernails, arched or curved

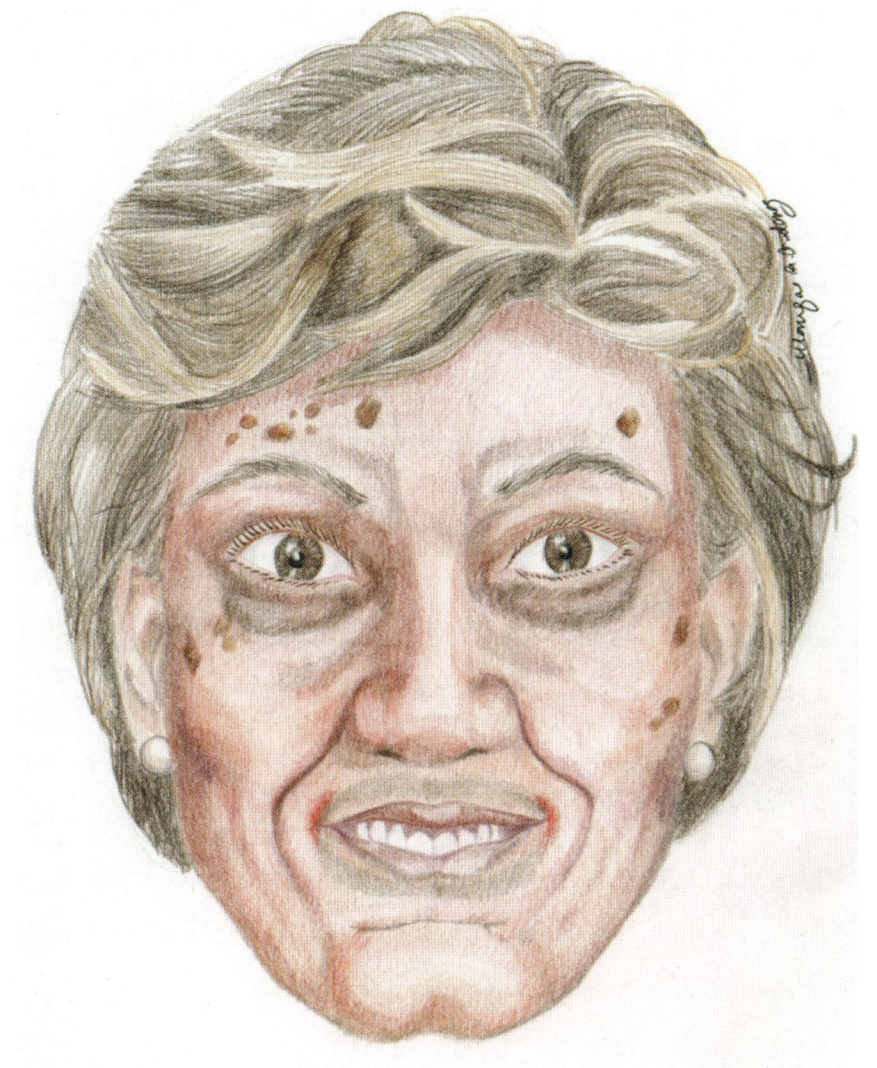

Colon Herbs

Colon herbs are best used in combination. Adjust herb amounts as needed. A combination might be a total of 1 heaping teaspoon three times a day or 4 capsules 3 times a day. It depends on your needs.

Colon Tonic herbs

Burdock root for colon, skin, and liver conditions.
Dandelion root improves bile output through stimulating the liver.
Red clover blossoms commonly used as a blood purifier.

Colon Anti-inflammatory herbs

Calendula flowers have liver and colon health benefits, as well as for leaky gut.
Chamomile flowers also stimulate digestion and release gas, as well relieving pain.
Marshmallow root is cooling and calms the colon from irritation.
White willow bark also relieves pain and settles the stomach.

Colon Diarrhea herbs (astringent)

White oak bark is the most common to slow excessive diarrhea, medium strength.
Shepherd's purse is the strongest and helps on excessive menstruation or other bleeding.
Red raspberry leaves also strengthen the uterus.

Colon Constipation herbs (stimulate colon peristalsis)

Cascara sagrada bark is a medium-strength laxative, safe but may cause some dependence.
Rhubarb root has the ability to normalize colon function, for too much or too little.
Yellow dock is a mild laxative which also helps with iron absorption.

Colon Spasm herbs

Cramp bark for smooth muscle tissue, including menstrual and leg cramps,

Lemon balm, is also a nerve restorative, helps thyroid, heart palpitations and anxiety.

Peppermint leaves also relieves gas and bloating.

Valerian root is useful for sleep and is a nerve tonic.

Colon Gas and Bloating herbs (carminatives)

Anise seeds chewed or swallowed release gas and bloating.

Caraway seeds chewed or swallowed release gas and bloating.

Chamomile flowers are also anti-inflammatory and for pain

Fennel seeds chewed or swallowed release gas and bloating.

Colon Leaky Gut regenerating herbs

Calendula flowers also help the liver. Bacteria can't grow in its presence.

Gotu kola leaves are also good for brain and memory function.

Plantain leaves for wound healing internally and externally.

Yarrow is a wound healer as well as beneficial for circulation.

Colon Homeopathic Medicine

Colon Situational Homeopathics

DRY constipation: Alum, Bry, Nat Mur

INACTIVE bowels: Alum, Caust, OP Plb

LARGE STOOLS: Nux Vom, children: Calc Carb, Collinsonia

OVERWEIGHT: Graphites, Calc Carb

Incontinence of stool: Aloe Socotrina

SPASMODIC: Nux Vom, Plb

Neurological: Alum, Plb

Hormonal: Sepia

Constipation Homeopathics

Aesculus Hip: sacroiliac/pelvic displacement pain with constipation, as if rectum full of sticks.

Aloe Socotrina: constipation alternates with incontinence of stool. Diarrhea sudden, can't make it to the bathroom.

Aluminum: severe constipation, dryness, mucus. Elderly, sedentary person. Travelers' constipation; defecation requires much exertion, with little results or a small amount of soft stool.

Bellis Perennis: painful (similar to Sepia); worsened after abdominal surgery or trauma to pelvic area. It is the arnica of the deeper tissues and organs.

Bryonia: a degree less than Aluminum. Dryness; associated with headaches; tension headache in forehead or occiput; tearing pain upon movement.

Calc Carb: overweight, especially children. Pass large stools, moaning and groaning. Happier with constipation (Phos Acid), than with diarrhea.

Calendula: for rectal tears from stools.

Causticum: similar to Nat Mur; history of straining, child not using bathroom. Cerebral override like Nat Mur, but worse to paralysis like MS. Burning and pressing pains.

Collinsonia: obstinate constipation, painful hemorrhoids, sensation of rectum full of sticks. Large bulky stools, incomplete emptying (Nux), intense heat and itching of anus.

Graphites: Overweight; anal fissures with knotty stools with mucus.

Kali Carb: hot poker up the rectum.

Natrum Mur: dry chronic of Bryonia with introverted psychological symptoms. Hold their stool, can't use someone else's bathroom, suppress the urge. Child afraid to ask – fear of being embarrassed or rejected; fear of bad odors offending others.

Nux Vomica: painful, cramps, spasms, addicted to laxatives. Nothing happens or sensation that stool slips back into rectum: reverse peristalsis sensation. Stools large. Sedentary living and poor diet.

Phosphorus: paralysis of area due to anesthesia or hemorrhoidectomy. Stools long and thin.

Plumbum: painful, spasmotic (Nux), inactivity (Alum); colic during pregnancy. Neurological problems; severe spasms.

Rhatania: sensation of glass-up-the-rectum.

Sepia: hormonal constipation with pregnancy; PMS. Weak bowel tone – sedentary life; better with exercise. Ineffectual urging, pain and bearing down. After pelvic surgery, when that area becomes weak: bladder incontinence; sensation of a ball or lump on sitting; rectum prolapsed w/hemorrhoids.

Diarrhea Homeopathics by Dr. Robin Murphy

Arsenicum album: food poisoning, bad water, antibiotics. Child diarrhea, dark green mucussy or brown black watery diarrhea. Epidemics or flu, especially stomach. Excoriating, burning, weakness and fainting, thirsty but sips a little; made worse by anything cold, better by warm drinks.

Carbo veg: light colored watery stools, offensive smelling, gas. Cholera, dysentery. Carbo Veg upper gas, China lower gas.

Chamomile: green, watery diarrhea, diarrhea during teething. Rotten egg odor or sulphury.

Cinchona: epidemic diarrhea, cholera. Dehydration. Great weakness, bloating lower intestine; drinks little and often. If doesn't work: China Ars or China Sulf.

Gelsemium: epidemic flu, stools brown watery; weaker after stools.

Mag carb: sour smelling stools, esp. children. Fever, sweat, sour vomiting.

Phosphoric acid: painless diarrhea, happy with diarrhea; apathetic. Emaciation, weakness.

Podophyllum: painless diarrhea, colic, profuse watery stools, looks like cornmeal, yellow mucus. Prolapsed anus, worse hot weather and in the morning.

Rheum: sour smelling brown stools with colic, painful urging; can't wash off the smell.

Sulphur (follows Arsenicum): rotten egg smell, yellow brown; suppressed skin problems.

Note: Use olive oil on skin to prevent dehydration.

Hemorrhoid Homeopathics

Aesculus: purplish color; rectal pains as if full of sticks. Pain worsened by standing, walking, sitting; better kneeling down. Itching, dryness, pulsating pain in pelvis/SI joint. Aggravated one hour after stools.

Aloe: purplish-grapelike.

Collinsonia: painful-bleeding, worsened by stool; sense of constriction.

Hamamelis: sore, bruised feeling. Use as tincture, ointment, suppositories.

Nux vomica: hangovers, indigestion, aggravated by alcohol with constipation. Often heavy drinker with hemorrhoids.

Peony: worms; peri-anal ulceration with sores and cracks; oozing w/offensive discharge. Anus feels swollen. Tearing pain before and after stool.

Rhatania: cutting, burning, sharp pain with anal fissures (nit ac, graph, rhat); broken glass feeling in anus, which also feels constricted. Made better with cold sitz baths.

Sepia: Pregnancy rectal prolapse; not well since abdominal surgery, childbirth.

Sulphur: burning, itching, Worsened with heat, bathing, alcohol.

Colon Cell Salts (including Constipation, Diarrhea, Hemorrhoids)

Constipation Cell Salts

Calc sulph: with fever, difficult breathing.

Ferr phos: constipation from weak peristalsis.

Kali mur: light colored stool.

Kali sulph: with hemorrhoids, offensive large stools.

Nat mur: from grief, inactivity, alternate days.

Mag phos: rheumatic, with gas, indigestion, infants.

Diarrhea Cell Salts

Calc phos: diarrhea with pus, gas, flakes, fistula.

Calc sulph: diarrhea of children. With pus and/or blood. Worsened by change of weather. Abscesses, fistula.

Ferr phos: at night, in summer, with red face, chronic.

Kali mur: from fatty foods.

Kali phos: diarrhea putrid smell, from fright with depression, brain fatigue, at night, after eating.

Mag phos: watery diarrhea, vomiting, cramp in calves, loose, watery, spasms.

Nat mur: chronic painless diarrhea, watery, abdominal pain, diarrhea after menses.

Nat phos: greenish diarrhea, itching, parasites.

Silicea: cadaver odor, diarrhea after milk.

Hemorrhoids Cell Salts

Calc fluor: sluggish, bleeding hemorrhoids, internal hemorrhoids, pain in back.

Calc phos: oozing fluid, painful, itchy, burning, with yellow pus.

Ferr phos: hemorrhoids with constipation, mucus of stomach, bowels.

Kali phos: rectum worse from constipation.

Mag phos: cutting, darting, lightning-like pain. Itches, scratching.

Nat mur: stinging, tearing pain, sore after stool.

Silicea: painful, hemorrhoids protrude during stool, lump in anus; in menses, parasites.

Aging

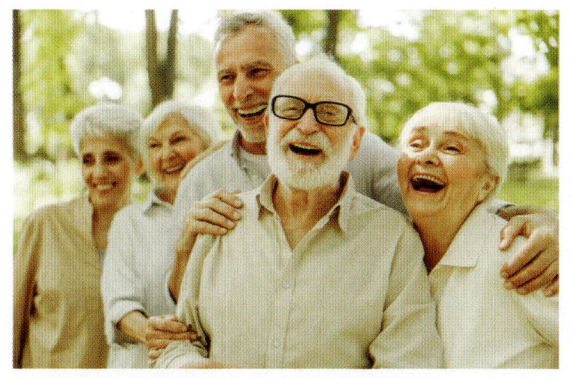

Aging is a complex set of circumstances. It has been said that it is the slow decay of body and mind until the end.

A great deal of fear can be associated with aging; for women it starts at menopause when the child-bearing years are done, with fear that beauty leaves, and sickness and loneliness takes over. Men may fear that they may be useless and lose their minds.

The ravages of aging may be put off when we take care of ourselves. We can look good, feel great, and have superb health if we can have a good diet, physical and mental exercise and use of the right supplements.

Common aging signs

- Sleep issues
- Heart disease
- Osteoporosis
- Hair loss
- Memory loss
- Alzheimer's
- Arthritis
- Diabetes
- Drug induced side effects
- Varicose veins
- Prostatitis
- Sagging
- Wrinkles

Aging Emotions

From **Feelings Buried Alive Never Die** by Karol Truman or **Heal Your Body** by Louise Hay:

Aging is about:
- Social beliefs
- Old thinking
- Fear of being one's self
- Inability to accept now, rejection of the now
- Long standing unresolved negative feelings

Aging Facial Diagnosis

Gray hair and eyebrows

Brown pigmentation on face and hands

Hairy ears

Zigzag veins on temples

Spider veins on eyelids

Eyes, gray or white half circle on the rim of the eyeball (arcus senilis)

Hairy nose (males)

Double chin

Other Signs

Neck wrinkles

Flat warts on abdomen

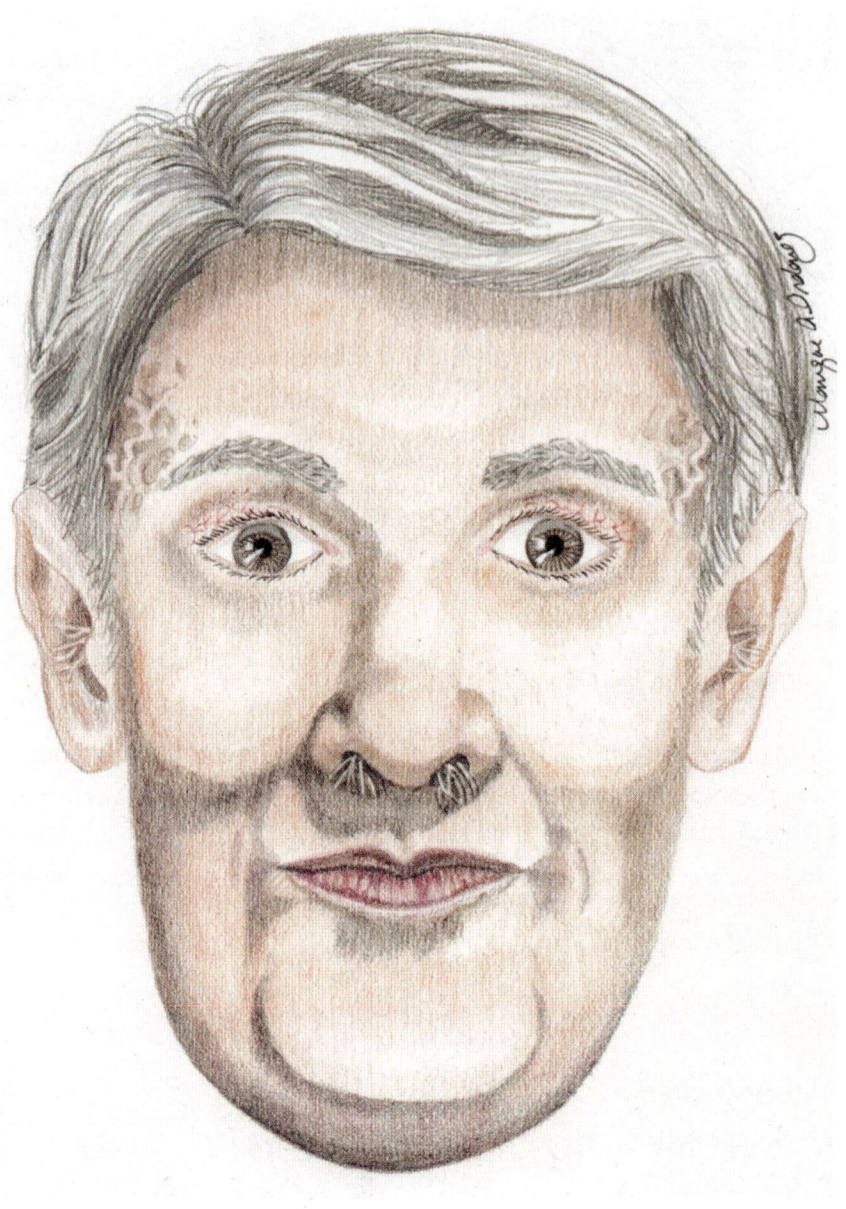

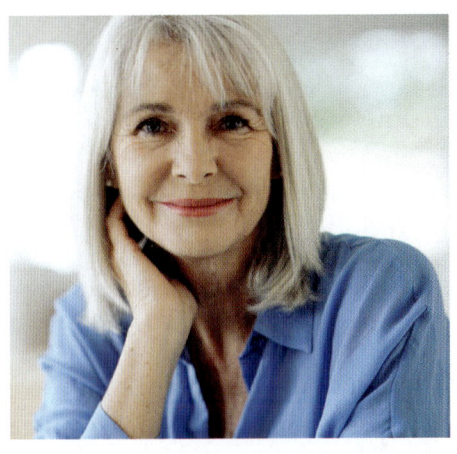

Prevention always keeps us in great shape and prevents disease and debilitating conditions.

Four Nasty Medications (Bad Boys)
1. High blood pressure meds
2. Cholesterol meds
3. Stomach acid reducers
4. Allergy meds

Anti-Aging Strategy

Aging References
DavesHealingNotes.com
Alzheimer's
Dementia
Insomnia
Incontinence
Prostate problems

Nutrition

Stage 1: eliminate the 4 bad boys.

Stage 2: adding antioxidants

Stage 3: Mucusless diet by Dr. Christopher

Medications (fewer medications lead to better health)

Stage 1: eliminate over the counter drugs, use homeopathic or herbals.

Stage 2: eliminate prescription drugs, using your doctor.

Exercise 30 minutes continuous, 3 times a week, minimum. It is important to keep moving with some sort of exercise that helps circulation, the brain, and other organ and joint function. One may start with a small daily walk of 10 minutes. Swimming is best as cardiovascular and weight-bearing exercise. All exercise helps to prevent osteoporosis, joint problems, and cardiovascular disease.

Attitude: meditate, pray, and consult with others you trust to be honest about you.

Stress: keep at a minimum by examining your lifestyle.

Purpose: question: Why are you here? Are you enjoying yourself?

Financial planning: are your finances working for you; are you planning ahead?

Spirituality: are you connecting with a higher power (two heads are better than one)?

Selfish versus selfless: are you fair to yourself, others, animals, or the environment?

Preventative Supplements

Salmon oil (health food store quality only): 4,000 mg a day for cardiovascular health

Grape seed extract: 200 mg per day for vein an antioxidant health

Greens: powders or capsules for cleansing and antioxidant properties to add to smoothie

Anti-Aging Herbs

These herbs protect the organs, are antioxidant, adaptogen, and anti-inflammatory.

Ashwagandha is an adaptogen for hormones, thyroid, inflammation, stress, energy.

Eleutherococcus is an adaptogens that helps with stress and energy.

Guggul helps with thyroid weakness and helps normalize cholesterol levels.

Rhodiola is an adaptogen, clears the mind, increases energy, strength.

Devil's claw is anti-inflammatory and helps joint health.

Hawthorn berry is gentle yet cardio-protective and also healing. May also help mild high blood pressure.

Anti-Aging Homeopathic Medicines

These are remedies that certain constitutional types may find helpful.

Aurum met: feels suicidal or deeply depressed, especially if forced to retire.

Calcarea phos: grumpy old person with digestive problems and osteoporosis.

Kali carb: black and white thinking with arthritic problems.

Lycopodium: low self-esteem, boaster, weakness and impotence in men. Feels worse 4 to 8 pm.

Selenium: weakness and low sexual function with greasy skin in men.

Silicea: weakened and delicate, shy, poor fingernails, scars easily.

Sulphur: the philosopher who reads a lot, outgoing, leader, skin problems.

Anti-Aging Cell Salts

Aging is potentiated by not having enough minerals and nutrients to maintain healthy cells. Cell salts can be helpful to prevent premature aging by supplying the cells with optimal mineral supplies. Use one to three remedies on a consistent basis for weakness, to slow the aging process, or stay healthy longer. **Note: diet is crucial to overall health.**

Calc phos: bone integrity.

Ferr phos: iron integrity, as needed.

Kali mur: lung health.

Kali phos: nervous system integrity, emotional health.

Mag phos: heart and muscle health.

Nat mur: emotional health, grieving.

Nat phos: digestive health.

Silicea: physically weak, overly shy.

Men's Health: Prostate

Men's health is often a neglected issue, as men normally don't look after their own health. We can't help it, we're men; that's just the way we are, we don't apologize. So, typically, men don't go to any healthcare professional unless something is really wrong with them.

The prostate is a small gland that surrounds the urethra in the pelvis cavity of males. It is normally the size of a walnut. Its job is to produce prostatic fluid that nourishes the sperm in an ejaculation. It is influenced by testosterone (large amounts) and progesterone and estrogen (small amounts).

Problems with the prostate include BPH (enlarged prostate), prostatitis (inflammation), erectile dysfunction, and even prostate cancer.

The three biggest issues for men: **BPH** (benign prostate hypertrophy) where the prostate swells and affects urination and sleep. It usually affects most men at some time over the age of 50. **Prostatitis** is inflammation of the prostate and can be related to BPH. This can result in urinary problems as well as pain. The third is probably the most common, **erectile dysfunction** (see DavesHealingNotes.com for more information). **Prostate cancer** is a less common issue, although certainly not unimportant.

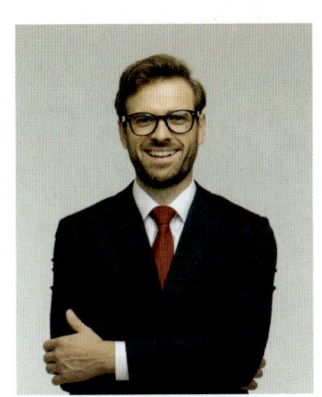

A happy health man is a joy to be around. Just ask my wife. Let's talk about three specific issues for men—prostate problems, sexual health, and energy matters.

When working well, the prostate goes unnoticed. As problems begin, so does frequent urination, irritation, and cancer becomes possible. You may notice difficulty in starting or stopping urination, dribbling, or weak urination. Prevention is always your best bet.

Dietary changes are not always easy, but they are very effective. Stay away from fats. Use 2 heaping tablespoons of ground flax a day. Stop smoking, give up alcohol, stay away from coffee, black tea, and soda pop. If you do not, prostate health may be a challenge. Most people I see for nutritional advice have a few of the above vices, but report back to me their tremendous boost in health, fitness and well-being after letting go of their habits. Making changes for your own health beats the alternative (treatments, surgery, medications with their side effects, etc.)

Getting up several times a night to urinate is a good sign you might have BPH (non-cancerous enlarged prostate). Several studies indicate Saw Palmetto works as effectively as some of the prescription medications, without the side effects. (Check with your doctor.)

Pain of the prostate, stemming from inflammation, can be localized or radiate to the pelvis, above the pubic bone, in the perineum, and upper thighs. There can be fever and chills, urging to urinate, as well as frequent and painful urination. Urinary retention can permanently damage the bladder. See your doctor if:

- You can't empty the bladder
- Blood in the urine
- Frequent urinary tract infections
- Bladder stones

Enlarged Prostate Symptoms

Because of the narrowed urethra, the body has to become more forceful in pushing urine through the body. The size of the prostate does not always determine how severe the obstruction or symptoms may be. Some men with greatly enlarged glands have little obstruction and few symptoms while others, whose glands are less enlarged, have more blockage and greater problems. Some men may not know they have a problem until they have acute urinary retention (Inability to urinate).

Common symptoms of BPH include:

- Weak or split stream of urine
- Hesitant, interrupted, weak stream
- Difficulty starting urination
- Dribbling of urine, especially after urinating
- Sense of not fully emptying the bladder
- Leaking of urine; incontinence
- Frequent urination and a strong/sudden desire to urinate, especially at night
- Urgency to urinate
- Night urination, getting up frequently
- Urinary stream that starts and stops
- Straining to urinate
- Returning to urinate again minutes after finishing
- Incomplete emptying of the bladder

Men who have had long-standing BPH with a gradual increase in symptoms may develop:

- Sudden inability to urinate
- Urinary tract infections
- Urinary stones
- Damage to the kidneys
- Blood in the urine

Prostate Emotions

From ***Feelings Buried Alive Never Die*** by Karol Truman or ***Heal Your Body*** by Louise Hay:

Prostate represents the masculine principle

Prostate problems:
- Belief in aging
- Feeling you are a victim
- Giving up
- Ideas are in conflict about sex
- Mental fears weaken the masculinity
- Refusing to let go of the past
- Sexual pressure and guilt

Prostate cancer:
- Repressed anger at being restricted

> "I hope I shall possess firmness and virtue enough to maintain what I consider the most enviable of all titles, the character of an honest man."
> —George Washington

Prostate Facial Diagnosis

Receding thinning hair

Too much hair growth on entrance of ear canal

Lower eyelids swollen, rosy red colored

Thick lower lip

Deficient hair growth in beard

Chin cleft, prominent

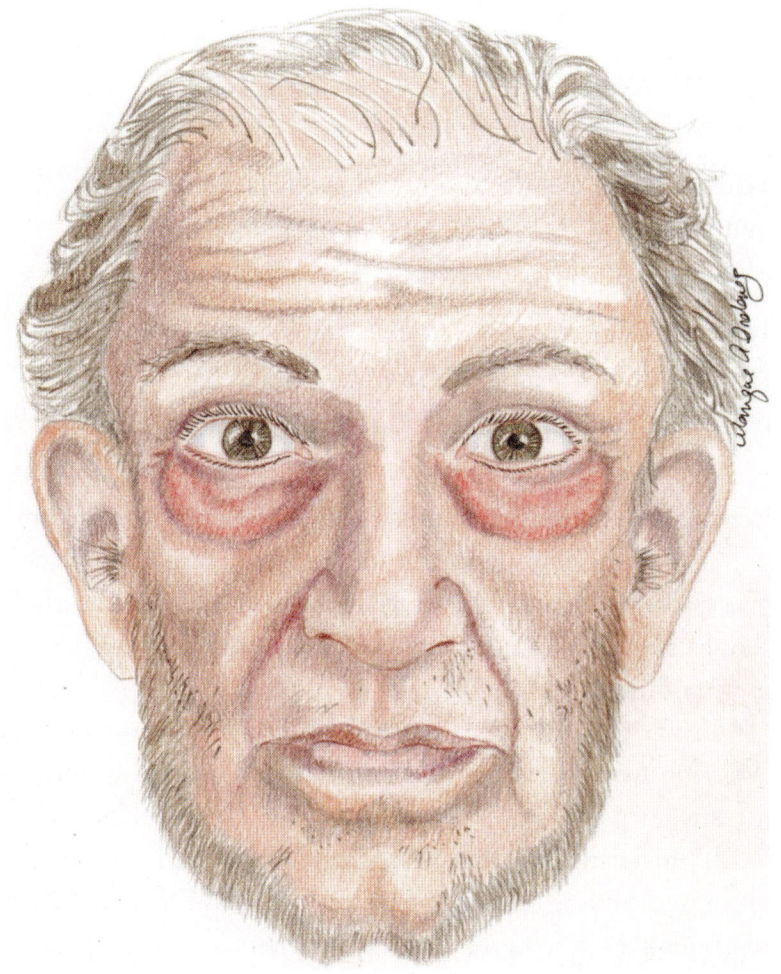

Prostate Nutrition

Zinc 50 mg a day for general prostate health

Selenium 100 mcg a day for prostate problems

Vitamin E 400 I.U. a day for genital health

Dietary restrictions: stay away from tobacco, alcohol, coffee, soda pop, processed foods as well as fast foods.

Herbs for Prostate

Prostate herbs help normalize testosterone, increase sexual energy, and sexual health.

Catuaba was used in South America for sexual vigor and male energy and motivation.

Damiana is helpful to reduce tension and build the nerves.

Ginseng root was used in ancient China for virility, longevity, and as an adaptogen to balance energy and stress conditions.

Ho Shuo Wu root in China is considered to increase longevity and virility.

Muira Puama also from South America called "potency wood" to enliven and improve male vigor.

Nettle root has been used for hair loss, prostate inflammation, and reduce testosterone loss.

Sarsaparilla has been used to enhance male potency and hormone production.

Tongkat ali is an exotic herb with a reputation for male vigor and stamina.

Tribulus has been used by many cultures to support healthy male virility, stamina and energy. May help the body to produce testosterone.

Herbs for Prostatitis

Excerpt from an article by Jacob Randall McKinney, T.H.

When the prostate is inflamed or swollen, it pinches the urethra which causes the difficulty in urination. Diuretics help prevent a buildup of excess urine in the bladder. **Hydrangea, Cleavers, Couch grass, Corn silk and Marshmallow** can be soothing to the area and relieve the bladder. These herbs should be taken in conjunction with plenty of pure, spring water. This will keep the bladder and urethra flushed.

Urinary system antimicrobials should be taken to support the urinary tract and to prevent any infection from spreading to the kidneys. **Uva Ursi, Goldenseal** or **Oregon grape root** are excellent for this purpose.

If prostatitis is a chronic condition, an overall, general weakness may be the problem and a deeper immune-building program may be required. **Siberian Ginseng, Astragalus, Echinacea** along with reproductive tonic herbs such as **Damiana** and **Sarsaparilla** are good additions.

Herbs for Painful Urination (see also Kidneys)

Corn silk soothes painful urination.

Marshmallow Root soothes mucus membranes and urethra.

Herbs to increase urine (diuretic)

Couch grass increases urinary output.

Dandelion leaf increases urinary output.

Herbs for Urinary Tract Infections

Cranberry extract inhibits bacterial colonization.

Echinacea reduces inflammation, stimulates the immune system, stimulates white cell production, and kills certain bacteria.

Oregon grape root is an herbal antibiotic, tonic, anti-microbial.

Pipsissawa is anti-microbial and used for short periods of time.

Uva Ursi is a urinary antiseptic for short term use.

Herbs for Muscle Spasms

Butterbur is antispasmodic, relaxes smooth muscle spasms and bladder spasms.

Kava reduces spasms but contraindicated for those on antidepressants, anti-anxiety, and sedative medications.

Prostate Homeopathic Medicines

Berberis vulgaris: pressure in pelvis; kidney and bladder inflammation with hematuria. Pain with urination. Uric acid diathesis. Kidney and back pain as if the back was broken.

Bryonia: urination frequent with hot, beer-colored urine.

Chimaphila umbellata: prostate hypertrophy, chronic bladder infection with prostatitis. Bladder and kidney pelvic mucus. Diuretic.

Echinacea ang: to fortify the immune system.

Equisetum: burning pain at the end of urination. Incontinence with elderly women, often combined with stool incontinence.

Pareira Brava: inflammation of the urinary tract. Colic pain and prostate enlargement. Pain and pressure in the upper shank; can urinate only on the knees. Relaxation of the smooth muscles.

Pulsatilla: frequent bladder pressure lying down; regular cramps. Inflammation of the genital organs. Bladder pains after urination.

Rhododendron: pain with urination. Joint and muscle pain, testes swollen and inflamed. Pinching discomfort.

Sabal serrulata: urinary incontinence, bladder mucus with or without prostate edema. Early symptoms of prostate enlargement.

Thuja: urinary disturbances, bladder inflammation, split-stream urination.

Prostate Cell Salts

Nat sulph: enlarged prostate with pus and mucus in urine.

Silicea: prostate enlargement. Discharge of prostate fluid when straining at stool.

Prostate References

Books

Homeopathy Now
by David R. Card

DavesHealingNotes.com
Prostate, BPH
Erectile Dysfunction

Women's Health: Child-Bearing Years Through Menopause

Some of the health challenges faced by women include hormonal issues, anxiety, mood swings, depression, infertility, lowered sex drive, insomnia, and crying spells. And that doesn't even cover the physical stuff like breast tenderness, cramping, bloating, sugar cravings, heavy bleeding, and vaginal discharges. Although many of these symptoms are hardly exclusive to women, they are not "normal" in any case.

From a natural perspective, most of these symptoms are the result of chemical pollution caused by either birth control devices or the standard American diet, rich in animal steroids, hormones, and fat. Such pollution disrupts estrogen receptors and contributes to **hormonal imbalances**.

Here we will cover PMS, Menstrual Cramping, and Infertility. Menopause comes later.

PMS symptoms may occur before or during a woman's period. Symptoms may include:

- Weight gain or bloating
- Moodiness, anxiety or depression
- Hormonal headaches
- Backaches, cramps
- Breast tenderness
- Difficulty concentrating or memory loss
- Loss of interest in usual activities
- Sugar and food cravings

PMS is associated with women's hormonal health. The menstrual cycle is normally 28 to 30 days long and symptoms often show up a week before menstrual bleeding. Some symptoms may last all month long. Woman may also experience frigidity, the lack of sexual interest.

A diet rich in animal fats and fast food may contribute to poor hormonal health. Other symptoms are caused by chemical hormone therapies, including birth control methods.

Natural remedies for PMS like herbs, cell salts and homeopathy, combined with a change of diet and the removal of chemical hormones, can be very helpful.

Hormone Emotions

From **Feelings Buried Alive Never Die** by Karol Truman or **Heal Your Body** by Louise Hay:

Female Problems:
- Emotional block where one's own sexuality is concerned
- Feeling inadequate in sexual role
- Feelings of fear or guilt about sex
- Refusing to let go of the past
- Rejecting female nature
- Emotional block where mate is concerned
- Menstrual problems
- Unresolved feelings of guilt
- Fears role as a woman
- Feels no joy in being a woman

Amenorrhea – no period: not wanting to be a woman, dislike of self

Dysmenorrhea – painful periods: dislike of self, hatred of the body or of women.

Fibroid tumors or cysts: nourishing a hurt from a a blow to the female ego.

Leucorrhea – female discharge: belief women are powerless over the opposite sex, anger at a male.

Menstrual problems: rejections of femininity, guilt, fear, belief that genitals are sinful or dirty.

Vaginitis: anger at mate, sexual guilt, punishing the self.

> After all those years as a woman hearing 'not thin enough, not pretty enough, not smart enough, not this enough, not that enough,' almost overnight I woke up one morning and thought, 'I'm enough.'
> —Anna Quindlen

Female Hormone Facial Diagnosis

Dark blond or brunettes

Freckles or brown spots on forehead – uterine fibroids

Bushy eyebrows – weak ovaries

Eyelashes fallen out – ovarian problems or extreme toxicity

Raw nasal opening – genital disturbance

Clear thin nasal discharge

Horizontal line above upper lip – weak ovaries and low sex drive

Prominent large lower lip – uterine and bladder weakness

Thickening under lower lips by corner of the mouth

Chronic acne of the chin area – hormonal disorders or uterine disease

Chin part – uterine hint

Fibroma (skin tag) – uterine fibroids

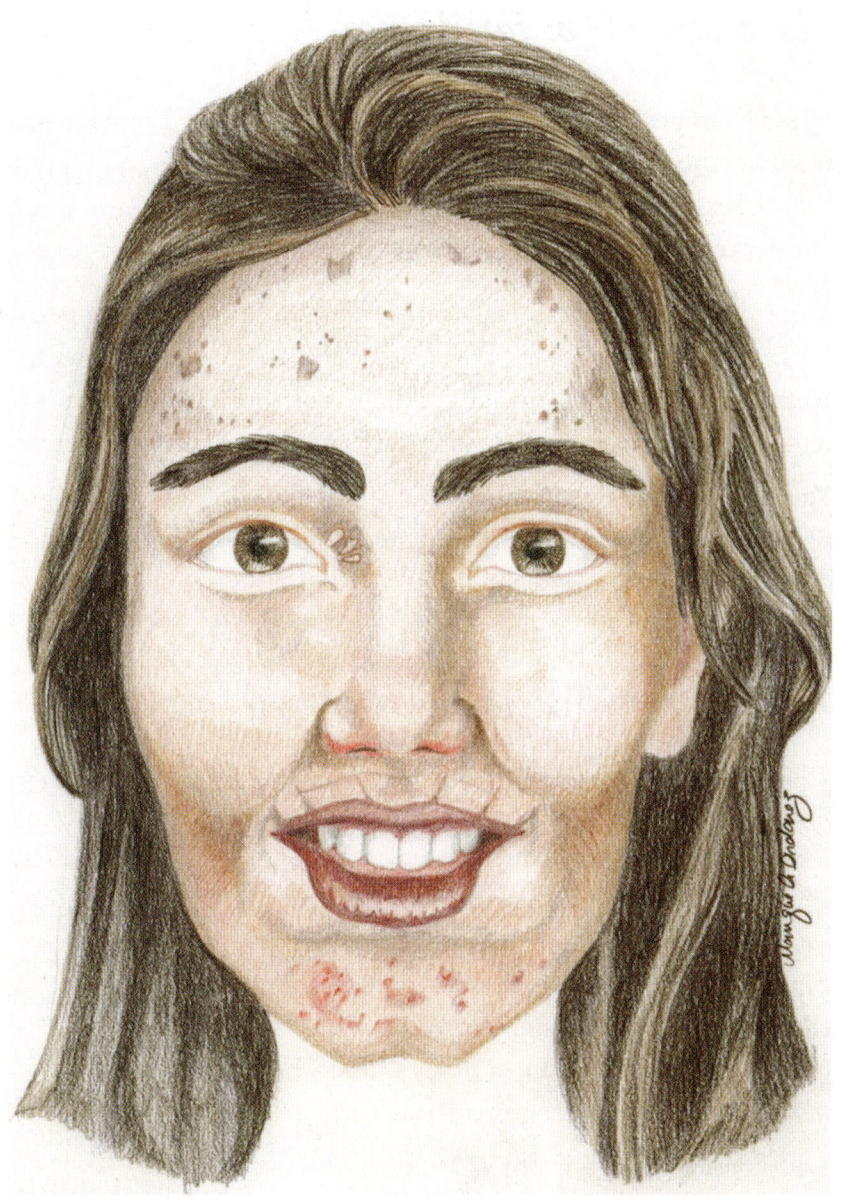

Hormone Herbs for Women

Vitex is progesterone promoting, useful for women who cry easily. A recent study showed that Vitex works as well as Prozac as an antidepressant; promotes fertility.

Blessed thistle regulates the hormones by its effect on estrogen metabolism in the liver.

Red raspberry is a detoxifier and helps to regulate hormones. Safe during pregnancy.

Yarrow has been used for centuries to help pelvic circulation and is known to enhance digestion and wound healing.

Licorice soothes the mucus membranes.

Red raspberry leaves have been used by Native Americans to strengthen the uterus and enhance iron absorption.

White peony is used in traditional Chinese medicine to build the blood when there is a weak uterus. It is used traditionally to help deal with uterine fibroids.

Dong quai is used in Chinese medicine to build the blood and enhance uterine circulation.

PMS (Premenstrual Syndrome) Herbs

Progesterone-increasing herbs for better balance with high estrogen:

Vitex (Chaste berry) reduces stress, reduces FSH (follicle stimulating hormone), reduces excess estrogen, controls hypothalamus-pituitary activity, influences the thyroid, calms the central nervous system and helps normalize dopamine action. The most general PMS herb, it's used to increase progesterone.

Lady's mantle herb is not as strong as Vitex for progesterone effect; also improves liver function and is a pelvic decongestant.

Yarrow is a pelvic decongestant, anti-inflammatory with progesterone-enhancing effect; calms the central nervous system.

Stress reducing herbs

Lavender is a pelvic decongestant, reduces urinary spasms, antibacterial, central nervous system sedative, digestive.

Melissa, lemon balm, to calm anxiety, heart palpitations, digestive problems.

Liver herbs that detoxify the body and help balance hormones:

Dandelion root reduces allergies, improves liver and kidney function, increases bile, reduces constipation, and is diuretic.

Milk thistle is a liver protector that helps it create more bile. Also a circulatory tonic.

Nutrition for colon health (constipation increases pelvic stagnation/toxicity in the system):

Psyllium husk – to create a bulking effect and reduce constipation.

Magnesium – increases absorption of water in the bowel and relaxes overtight muscles.

Menstrual Cramping Herbs

One type of menstrual cramps is caused by uterine contractions that are too strong and occur too frequently. Between contractions the muscles do not relax properly. This reduces blood circulation throughout the uterus muscles which creates pain.

The second type of menstrual cramps is due to an inflammation of the pelvis. This inflammation can be due to misalignment of the uterus, uterine fibroids, or endometriosis. Usually this type of cramping occurs later in life and gets worse with age.

Other common symptoms that can accompany cramping include: low back pain, nausea, diarrhea, headaches, fatigue, abdominal bloating, vomiting, and dizziness. **Herbs that can aid relief of cramps** include:

- Angelica
- Asparagus root
- Basil
- Bilberry
- Black cohosh
- Black haw
- Calendula
- Caraway
- Chamomile
- Cramp bark
- Dong quai
- False unicorn
- Ginger
- Guggul
- Hops
- Lemon balm
- Passion flower
- Peony root
- Red raspberry leaf
- Squaw vine
- Valerian
- White willow
- Wild yam
- Yarrow

Nutrition also plays a part in relief of menstrual cramps. Nutritional aids may include: fish oils, phenylalanine, calcium, magnesium, manganese, forskolin, vitamin B1, vitamin B3, vitamin B6, and vitamin E.

PMS Homeopathic Medicines

Calcarea carb (Puls): complex, heavy build; can't sleep from worry; anticipation, fear something bad will happen. Sensitive emotionally, worsened by watching sad movies, can't watch news on television, feels vulnerable. Cramps in feet or legs, edema (swelling, fluid retention), breasts swollen, tender and sore. Constipation before period; Increased desire for sweets.

Ignatia (associated with Natrum mur): mood changes, frustration, argumentative, looking for a fight. Premenstrual twitches or spasms in parts of the body. Bothered by odors; headaches. Problems with relationships, slighted easily, unrealistically idealistic. Holds in frustrations and hurts and remembers them. Hard on themselves, perfectionistic; guilt over not having done enough.

Lachesis: severe violent, abusive, jealous, loquacious. Manic-depressive, hypertensive, suspicious. Hot-blooded, hyper, can't sleep, everything is a party, shopping sprees, possible alcoholism. With menstrual flow, all is back to normal.

Pulsatilla: weepy, sad, feels abandoned, loves consolation, hard to please, contrary. Craves/binges on pastry and creamy foods, sad at sunset. Water retention, swelling, weight fluctuations at period. Scanty menses, feels better with normal flow; spots for several days. Headaches.

Sepia: irritable, depressed. Low sex drive, worsened by consolation. Wants to be left alone, exhaustion. Heaviness in back or uterus as if a weight. Constipated.

Menstrual Cramping Homeopathic Medicines

Menstrual cramps are the effect of the uterine lining sloughing off or the muscles of the uterus or cervix in spasm. It is also called dysmenorrhea or a painful period. Menstrual cramping is seen in younger women and improves with age. There are estimates of 7% to 15% with severe symptoms. It happens when a woman is not pregnant and is at the end of her cycle, when the estrogen and progesterone levels are low. Then prostaglandins cause the breakdown of the endometrial lining and is gotten rid of through the menstrual low.

Belladonna: colicky, throbbing pelvic pains and bad smelling, bright blood; hot feeling, dragging pains that radiate to the lumbar area; oversensitivity to movement, noise and light.

Caulophyllum: spasmodic pain, bearing-down pains, normal or scanty flow; sympathetic spasms in the bladder, rectum or bowels. In patients subject to rheumatism of the small joints.

Chamomila: neuralgic dysmenorrhea, drawing pain from the lower part of the back forward. Gripping, pinching, labor-like pains in uterus w/discharge of large blood clots; frequent desire to urinate. Excessive irritability and impatience.

Cimicifuga: severe pains down back, thighs, and hips, hysteric spasms, cramps, tenderness of lower abdomen. Rheumatism.

Cocculus: menstrual colic from gas in the intestines, distention of the abdomen; sharp, cramp-like pains; headache and nausea as in sea sickness. Scanty, irregular, painful flow.

Graphites: cramping with skin problems (eczema with honey-like discharges and scarring), menses too late, gushing acrid discharges, vagina too hot or cold; aversion to sex.

Mag phos: cramping pains especially before the bleeding begins and is strongest the first and second day. Blood is dark, person doubles over in pain, made better with local warmth.

Nux vomica: cramping with anger, irritability, rage, addictive behaviors, craving for stimulants. Digestive issues, menses irregular or too early. Pain, cramping in lower back causes person to double over; uterine spasms with blood clots.

Veratrum album: colicky pains, nausea and diarrhea; strong bleeding that is too early.

Viburnum opulus: strong pains in pelvic and lumbar areas, pain in vagina, radiating to thighs. Blood of pale color, or clumpy dark, or has membranous discharges. Period late or short duration; colic-type pains before the bleeding begins (pelvic migraine).

> **Hormone Cell Salts For Menstrual Cramping**
>
> Calc phos 6X – with severe backache
>
> Ferr phos 6X – inflammation
>
> Kali phos 6X – nerve pain (in back)
>
> Mag phos 6X – sharp cramping, better by heat

Hormones and Cell Salts

Calc fluor affects the connective tissue and is associated with breast lumps and tumors. It is used for prolapsed uterus. Heavy bearing-down pains in the pelvic area and thighs. Helps childbirth in frail women and also good for gas in pregnancy.

Calc phos at menstrual onset where it is slow in coming, too little or excessive. Egg-white consistency vaginal discharges. Prolapsed uterus; excessive sexual desire before the period.

Calc sulph for late menstrual period, long-lasting with headache. Thick white vaginal discharges and cutting or sharp pains of the right ovary.

Ferr phos for menses every three weeks. Bearing-down sensation and pain on top of the head. Vagina dry and hot. Vaginal irritation; pain during sex.

Kali mur in menstruation too late or suppressed, stopped or too early. Excessive discharges, dark-clotted or tough, black blood like tar. Vaginal discharges milky white mucus, thick, non-irritating, bland. Morning sickness with vomiting of white mucus.

Kali phos in menstruation too late or too scanty; in pale, irritable, sensitive women. Delayed menses with depression. Too profuse discharge, deep red or black-red, thin, with sometimes an offensive odor. Feeble and ineffectual labor pains. Offensive vaginal discharges. Periodical discharges of copious orange colored fluid from vagina and rectum. Sexual desire intense for days after menses.

Kali sulph in menses too late, scanty. Painful menses, with a feeling of weight in the abdomen. Vaginal discharge is yellowish and watery.

Hormones and Cell Salts continued...

Mag phos in menstrual pain before the flow. Menstrual cramps made better with heat and bending over, and flow. Flow is dark and fibrous and stringy. Painful period with discharge of membranes. Menses too early, dark, stringy, tarry, flowing at night leaving a stain. Swelling of external genitalia. Ovarian neuralgic pains. Vaginal irritation. Swollen labia at times intensely painful.

Nat mur with sexual aversion from dryness. Burning, smarting in vagina during sex. Infertility. Menses delayed from grief. Bearing-down pains, worse in the morning. Prolapsed uterus with aching in the lower back area. Feels hot during the period. White vaginal discharges that can turn green and can be acrid and have a watery appearance. Can have a thick white vaginal discharge instead of a period.

Nat phos in menses too early, pale, thin, and watery. During period the feet are ice cold in the morning and burn in bed at night. Infertility with acid secretion from vagina. Sour smelling discharges. Morning sickness with sour discharges. Vaginal discharges are sour, creamy, honey-colored, or acid and watery.

Nat sulph with nosebleed during menses which are acrid and profuse. Burning of the throat during menses. Herpes on vulva with inflammation. Vaginal discharge yellow-green from gonorrhea.

Silicea when menses is early. Watery discharge instead of menses. No menses for months. Spotting between periods. Increased menses with paroxysms of icy coldness over the whole body. Discharge of blood from vagina every time child is nursed. Cutting pains moving upwards in vagina, worsened by nursing. Vaginal cysts. Abscesses of the labia. Vaginal discharges that are milky, acrid, gushing, worse during urination. Sensitive, itching of vulva and vagina. Cutting pain around the navel with vaginal discharges. Miscarriage or infertility due to weakness. Nausea during sex. Sterility; excessive desire for sex.

Hormone References

Books

Seven Symbols of Healing, Homeopathy Today
by David R. Card

DavesHealingNotes.com

Amenorrhea
Endometriosis
Melisma
PCOS
PMS

Infertility

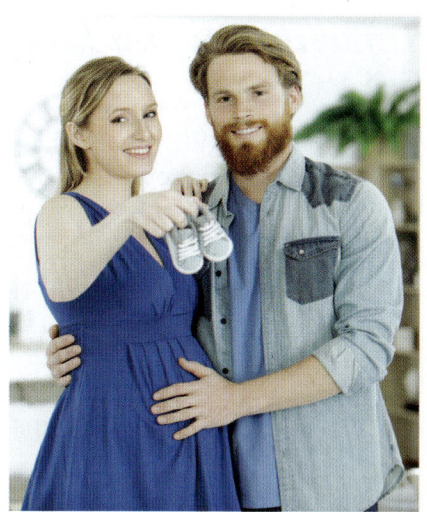

Infertility is the inability to conceive. Most women conceive within 12 months after intercourse, a smaller percentage in 24 months, and a few percent in 36 months. After 36 months, some intervention is usually taken.

There are structural problems that may impede the conception of a child. A woman's body may have blocked or scarred fallopian tubes, damage to the uterus, pelvic inflammatory diseases, hormone imbalances, endometriosis, polycycstic ovaries (PCOS), unfavorable age, or excessive weight. Stress can also be a factor, since it causes the fallopian tubes to contract.

For men, physical factors may include, low sperm count (often caused by environmental toxins), poor sperm quality, blockage of tubes carrying the seminal fluid from the testicles, and hormone imbalance.

The following items found inside the home can negatively affect fertility:
- Smoking or second hand smoke
- Household cleaners
- Pesticides, herbicides
- Microwave emissions
- Electric blankets or heating pads
- Hot tubs
- New carpet
- Varnish

In addition to all of the above conditions, it is important that both partners be in as healthy state as possible so conception can occur. Eating a diet high in essential fatty acids, fruits and vegetables, and fermented dairy are important for alkalizing the body so that the sperm is able to fertilize the egg.

Infertility Emotions

From ***Feelings Buried Alive Never Die*** by Karol Truman or ***Heal Your Body*** by Louise Hay:

Extreme nervous tension

Hard and cold attitudes

Fear and resistance to the process of life

Not needing to go through the parenting experience

Infertility Facial Diagnosis

Hair starts high on the forehead – hormone deficiency

Naturally thin eyebrows – estrogen deficiency

Extra thick eyebrows – excess testosterone

Cheeks hanging – ovarian signs

Upper lip vertical lines – estrogen deficiency

Upper lip hair – hormones disturbed

Chin hair with chronic acne – ovarian problems

Chin hair beard – hormonal imbalances

Lower lip exceptionally large – uterine weakness

Acne on chin – uterine weakness

Other body signs

Women with exceptionally long legs – ovarian problems

Tiny delicate women – ovarian problems

Large thighs – hormonal imbalance

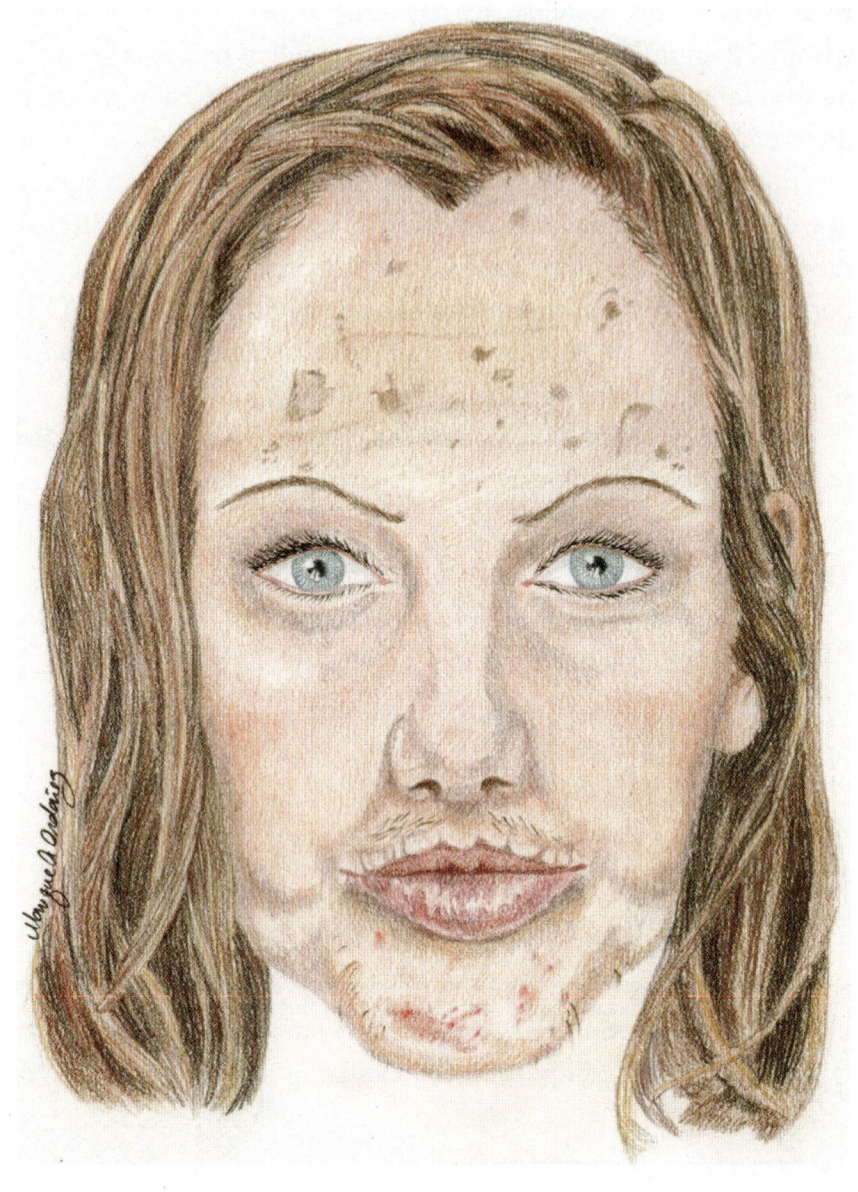

Infertility Herbs

Herbal medicine offers several body-balancing herbs which can lead to increased fertility. Many of them work to balance hormones and increase strength and vitality. Herbs can be taken individually or together in a formula. Herbs for women seeking better fertility include:

Ashwagandha supports the adrenals and thyroid, helps with stress and energy.

Kelp is for thyroid support. If the thyroid is not strong you can't hold the baby.

Panax Ginseng is for delicate tired women.

Saw Palmetto is for PCOS symptoms. See more below.

Shatavari is an Ayurvedic herb that helps with deficiency symptoms.

Vitex is progesterone promoting, useful for women who cry easily. A recent study showed that Vitex promotes fertility.

Infertility Homeopathic Medicines

#1 Natrum muriaticum: top remedy for grief and anxiety, which can suppress menses and create aversion to sex. Genital herpes, vaginal discharges acrid and watery.

Agnus castus: suppressed or scanty menses, no sexual desire; burned out sexually.

Aurum metallicum: severe depression, suicidal thoughts; financial worries. Uterus enlarged or prolapsed. Burning, smarting vulva; labia red, swollen.

Conium: bloating before menses; breasts enlarged, painful before and during menses; cervical problems, low sex drive, multiple sclerosis. Depression and poor concentration.

Natrum carb: oversensitivity, music makes her weep, resulting from depression. Menses painful, bearing down sensation. Weak digestion; can't tolerate milk. Discharges thick, yellow, ropy.

Sepia: depression with isolation, exhaustion, severe lack of sex drive. Never well since childbirth, onset of menses, or birth control pill usage. Uterine prolapse.

Infertility Cell Salts

Nat mur: vaginal dryness, aversion to sex (since grief). Possible genital herpes.

Nat phos: creamy, sour, acidic vaginal discharges.

Silicea: ice cold body, vaginal cysts. Nausea during sex.

Infertility References

Books

Seven Symbols of Healing, by David R. Card

DavesHealingNotes.com

Amenorrhea
PCOS

PCOS Herbs (Polycystic Ovarian Syndrome)

The most important herbs for PCOS are **Vitex** and **Saw palmetto** – use these in combination.

Vitex works on both PMS and fertility issues.

Saw palmetto is traditionally used for prostate problems in older men, but it also reduces androgens in women and improves urinary function.

Other herbs for polycystic ovarian syndrome:

Schizandra is an adaptogen that vitalizes the HPA axis as well as improving liver and respiratory function.

Ashwagandha is also an adaptogen and works similar to Schizandra but also supports thyroid.

Blue vervain is exceptional for those stressed women of executive skills and challenges. Many herbalists use this as their primary herb for menopausal hot flashes.

PCOS Homeopathic Medicines

#1 Sepia: facial hair, acne with menstruation, irregularity in period, masculine, hair loss on head, low sex drive, exhausted, obesity especially during menopause.

Calcarea carb: obesity, cold clammy feet, overworker, weak ankles, sweats at night, especially need the window open, fear of rodents, menopause problems, acne, possible hair loss, hoarse voice.

Graphites: obesity with skin problems such as eczema with yellow, honey-like discharges, tendency to keloids (ropy scarring), acne with menstrual irregularities.

Natrum mur: for those who are sensitive, isolate when needing protection, crave salty foods. Vaginal dryness, acne, hair loss, facial hair, low voice.

Thuja: with a tendency to warts (including genital) or other non-cancerous growths, acne. Facial hair as well as hair loss; feels guilty or unworthy, may have hoarse voice.

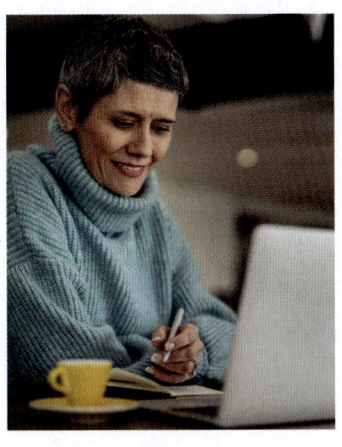

Menopause

Menopause starts, generally, between the age of 45 and 50. Sometimes it may start before 40 and last as long as 55. A woman's period becomes irregular, becoming less frequent, and will finally leave during this time. Or, women may have more frequent periods with heavier bleeding. In other cases the period becomes lighter and more watery, can become darker with clotty discharges, and can become mucus-like.

Also during this time the face grows round, the breasts sag. Others lose weight and severely wrinkle. The face gets more hair. The hair of the head thins, and the posture may droop. The uterus recedes, and the ovaries turn into connective tissue. Often the uterus sags; prolapse is common. This is why many women get hysterectomies. It is for this very reason you must not forget how important the care of your pelvic area is.

Hysterectomy

The removal of the uterus is called a hysterectomy. It may be removed because nature is not doing its job (or we are convinced of this). If a woman is under 50 years of age and has had a *partial* hysterectomy, that's good news because the ovaries can produce estrogen and progesterone at near normal levels until menopause comes on.

A full hysterectomy is the removal of the ovaries as well as the uterus and can be dealt with reasonably well. We can help nature by getting the adrenals to do their job by producing estrogen and progesterone and storing them in the fat cells—encouraged by using an adrenal formula.

The adrenals as hormone producers in menopause

When a woman loses her ovaries from surgery, the adrenals must take over and produce the hormones and store them in the fat cells of the body. (Super skinny women are at a disadvantage here.) The adrenals are glands that sit on top of the kidneys.

Hormone replacement vs natural treatment

Estrogen hormone replacement is popular because it produces fast results in treating hot flashes, vaginal thinning and dryness, and osteoporosis. It has also shown to improve emotional symptoms in some women. There is much controversy regarding its heart and cardiovascular benefits.

Considerable research shows that hormonal replacement therapy alters monthly cycles, causes cancer, liver disease, and increases risks of gallbladder disease. It has been shown to produce depression and promote or cause uterine fibroids. Interestingly, some research shows it causes cardiovascular diseases such as high blood pressure, heart attacks and even blood clots (strokes)!

The choice really comes down to knowing your options and being informed about them.

Progesterone replacement therapy with cream is also very popular with almost everyone, as it is touted as "natural." The fact is that there are no natural progesterone creams, *period*. They are derived from Wild Yam in a laboratory and come out as a chemical just like any other drug. By mouth or by skin it is a drug. Some studies show that it reduces the risks of uterine cancer.

But they also show that these creams can negatively affect cholesterol, blood sugar, blood pressure, and cardiovascular health. They also change the emotions and cause breast cancer. Remember, it is the game of cost versus benefit. Do you want to play the game? Even if these drugs may help you to feel better, there are three important risks:

1. They atrophy your glands. If you don't use them, you lose them.
2. They damage your feedback mechanisms (a constant bombardment of hormones may damage your receptors).
3. Cellular hormonal resistance is dead-ended and the cells no longer respond. (There's no natural ebb-and-flow of hormones.)

IF THESE PROBLEMS cause permanent damage, YOU MAY BE STUCK ON DRUGS UNTIL YOU DIE!

BIO-IDENTICAL doesn't mean natural, just drugs that are more specific. They are usually compounded at a special pharmacy and like all drugs can treat symptoms quickly. They have many of the same drawbacks as normal hormonal replacement therapy.

OK, OK, so now you have heard the bad news. **The good news is** – all you have to do is help your body work the way it is supposed to and nature will take away most of the symptoms of menopause!

Menopause Emotions

Menopause is a time of change in a woman's life when she can experience fears of getting old, abandonment, or getting sick.

From ***Feelings Buried Alive Never Die*** by Karol Truman or ***Heal Your Body*** by Louise Hay:

- Fears this time of life and getting older
- Fears of being rejected
- Feeling useless
- Fear of no longer being wanted
- Fear of aging
- Self-rejection
- Not feeling good enough

Menopause Facial Diagnosis

Hair on upper lip, chin and face

Skin tags, neck

Graying, thinning hair

Wrinkling sagging skin

Crying expression – an emotional face

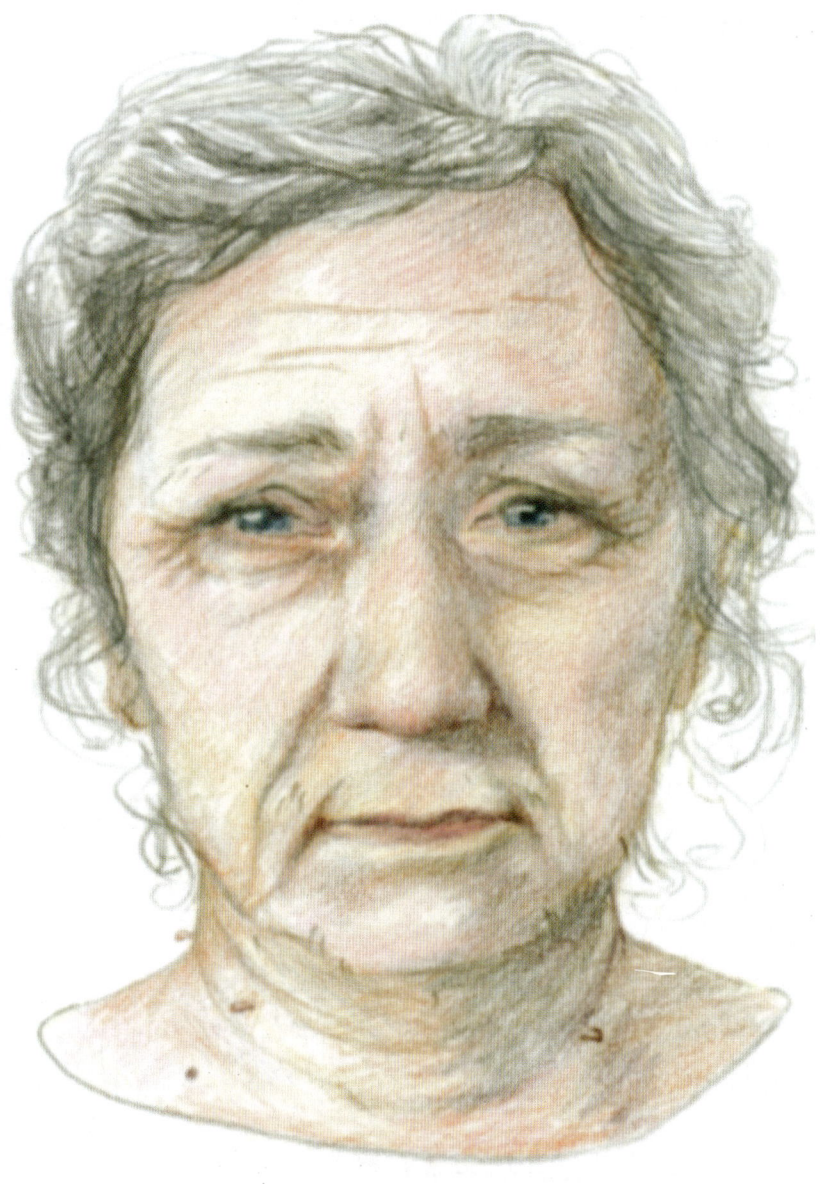

Menopause Herbs

Herbs have been used for thousands of years successfully to help ease women through menopause. Most herbs are safe and will not conflict with any other medications. Check with your doctor or other health care provider if in doubt. Use reasonable amounts for best results and safety. Use a total of 1 heaping teaspoon of single herbs or a combination as tea up to 3 times a day. If powdered, use 2 capsules 3 times a day.

Below is a list of single herbs to be used individually or your own combination:

Angelica archangelica: digestive support; respiratory, immune and liver support

Black Cohosh: for hot flashes, depression, vaginal dryness, PMS, irritability, fatigue.

Blessed Thistle: PMS, infertility, sweating, bloating, liver health, ulcers. Not for pregnancy.

Calendula: anti-inflammatory, wound healing, anti-bacterial, water retention.

Cayenne: circulation. Muscle and nerve pains. Shoulder-arm syndrome (numbness due to a lack of circulation). Spinal pains.

Chamomile: gas, bloating, anti-spasmodic, wound healing ability. Heals ulcers and has a calming effect. Menstrual cramps.

Damiana: depression, hormones, sex drive, energy.

Dandelion root: liver support, hormone conversion in the liver.

Dong Quai: hormonal balance, breast fibroids, PMS, menopause, liver, upper respiratory, cardiovascular, Raynaud's syndrome.

Eleutherococcus is an adaptogen which supports healthy adrenal and immune function. Healthy adrenals produce the right hormones for menopause.

Gingko: memory, concentration, depression, peripheral circulation. Meniere's disease, ringing in ears. Weak legs.

Ginseng (American, Chinese, or Korean): adaptogen, concentration, mood, cholesterol, diabetes, infrequent or ceased menstruation.

Hawthorn berries and leaves: improve circulation, digestive support, and connective tissue support. Heart tonic, lowers blood pressure. Useful for heart palpitations, and insomnia.

Lady's mantle: promotes progesterone. Pelvic health tonic for reducing symptoms of hemorrhoids and abnormal discharges.

Melissa (Lemon balm): calms heart palpitations and the nerves; stress, depression, anti-spasmodic, anti-viral, digestion, menstrual cramps.

Motherwort: heart, palpitations, lowers blood pressure, menstrual problems, PMS, menopause.

Passion flower: anxiety, insomnia, heart palpitations. Painful menstruation. Drug withdrawal, epilepsy, sedative.

Red Clover: menstrual regulation, estrogen-like effects, wound healing, regulates hot flashes, sweating, palpitations, depression.

Red Raspberry: hormonal balancing, colds and flu, herbal iron.

Sage leaf supports digestive health, estrogen production, hormone balance, and aids in decreasing symptoms of hot flashes.

Menopause Herbs continued…

Sarsaparilla: Balances hormones, blood purifiers, skin conditions, cholesterol, anti-inflammatory. Do not use during pregnancy.

Shepherd's Purse: excessive bleeding of any kind, especially for uterine fibroids. Also useful for digestive problems and hemorrhoids.

St. John's Wort: nervousness, stress, depression associated with hormones and menopause. It is also a fine anti-viral.

Suma: menopausal hormone symptoms such as hot flashes. Also for enhanced energy.

Uva Ursi: urinary tract infections and hormonal symptoms such as water retention.

Vitex: for PMS, depression, endometriosis. Normalizes estrogen and progesterone levels.

Yarrow: stops bleeding of any kind as well as helping the liver and gastrointestinal tract. It is also helpful for cystitis and painful periods. Fevers, in order to increase sweating.

Menopause Homeopathic Medicines

The following are the most frequently used homeopathics for menopause. See symptoms in individual remedies below. 3=most useful, 2=useful, 1=relatively useful.

Remedy	Breast Fibroids	Breast Cancer	Hair-Excess	Hair Loss	Heart Problems	Hot Flashes	Incontinence	Insomnia	Memory problems	Osteoporosis	Thyroid	Uterine bleeding	Uterine cancer	Uterine fibroids	Uterine polyps	Vaginal dryness
Aurum met				3	3	1		2	2			1	1		3	
Calc carb	2	1		2	2			3	2	2	3	3	2	3		3
Conium	3	3		2			1	2	2				3	2	2	
Gelsemium					1		2	2	2			1		1		
Glonoinum				1	1	2		2	2							
Graphites	2	3		3		2		2	2		1		1	3	2	2
Lachesis		2		3	3	2		3	2		2	3	3	2	2	
Manganum ace						2		1				1			1	
Natrum Mur			1	3	2		1	2	2		3	1	2	3	2	3
Platinum Met									3			3	1	3	1	
Psorinum		2		1	2	2		1	1			3			1	
Pulsatilla	1	1		1	3	2	2	3	1			3	1	1	3	
Sanguinaria		2				2		1				2	1	1	1	
Sepia	2	2	1	3		3	2	3	1	3	2	3	3	3	3	3
Sulphuricum Acid				1		2		1				1	1	1	1	
Tuberculinum	1	1		1		3		2	2			2		1	2	

Aurum met: flushes of blood to the heart and head, high blood pressure, bluish red face. Stress from financial problems, suicidal feeling.

Calc carb: obesity, cold damp feet, fears of bad news. Weak ankles. Menses heavy, early. Uterine polyps. Sweating itching burning in genital region. Milky yellow vaginal discharges. Heart palpitation.

Conium mac: Nervous exhaustion, circulatory disturbances, fear of being alone, trembling, cold sweat on the head, lower abdominal itching, sun sensitivity, uterine prolapse, effects from repressed sex. Breast fibroids, tumors, cancer. Stitching pains in nipples.

Menopause Homeopathic Medicines continued...

Gelsemium: fear getting up in front of groups, dull headaches. Heart problems, red face, cold hands and face. Headaches, rush of blood to head. Dizzy, shaken bruised feeling. Low back pains. Uterus feels squeezed. Sex painful from tight vaginal muscles. Weak heart sensation.

Glonoinum: High blood pressure, whole head pulsates, sudden hot flashes with sweating, dizziness, weakness, nausea.

Graphites: obesity, skin scars easily, or eczema with honey-like discharges. Constipation, light period, with corrosive white watery discharges. Menopausal depression. Crying, low self-esteem. Hot flashes start below and go up body. Sweating sour. Periods irregular, months apart. Exhausted, apathetic.

Lachesis: hot flashes and sweating, especially at night, with burning on top of the head. Can't stand anything around neck. Intense, talkative, jealous. Bipolar symptoms. Problems left-sided (ovary). Tight throat. Low or high blood pressure. Varicose veins. Craves stimulants. High sex drive. Uterine fibroids. Heart palpitations, insomnia. Profuse bleeding.

Manganum ace: Becomes sad and discouraged; anxiety and fear. Sudden heavy facial hot sweats and itch. Changes in the voice. Skin sore to touch. Parkinson's. Knee pains. Feels better lying down.

Natrum mur: feels depressed, isolates from grief. Craves salt. Skin dry; clear runny nose. Fever blisters. Genital herpes, low sex drive, dry burning sex. Uterine prolapse. Symptoms from disappointed love.

Platinum met: heavy painful periods. Constipation. Arrogant. Hypersexual. Painful, sensitive genitals. Menses too early, profuse with dark clots. Uterine prolapse, fibroids, cancer. Burning ovary pains.

Psorinum: hot flashes with sweating – feels as if warm water was poured over them. Menses early with heavy bleeding and weakness. Skin problems with intense itching. Painful periods nearing menopause.

Pulsatilla: fearful, whiny voice, wants to be held. Symptoms are changeable or alternate. Mucus conditions including sinus, bronchitis. Liver or gallbladder problems shown by an inability to tolerate fats. Varicose veins with inflammation. High sex drive from fear of abandonment.

Sanguinaria: right-sided sick migraines. Hot flashes start top of head to the bottom of body. Smelly vaginal discharges. Breasts painfully enlarged. Burning hands, feet, facial skin eruptions. Over-sensitivity, moody, facial redness. Heart palpitations. Arthritis. Irregular periods.

Sepia: anxiety felt in the chest, restless, moody. Anemia, headaches. Low sex drive. Voice changes, irritable and apathetic. Constipation, hemorrhoids. Uterine prolapse, must cross legs. Yells and screams at family; wants to be alone. Chronic eczema and psoriasis. Heart palpitations in the evening. Hot flashes day and night. Headaches in the left eye. Liver spots. Yellow saddle across the nose.

Sulphuricum acidum: feels great after the hot flashes are done. Dark bleeding; cervical erosion (like an open wound); vaginal and uterine prolapse. Hot flashes with tremors, facial sweating. Tremors and weakness.

Tuberculinum: hot flashes with sweating and tendency to chills. Breast tension and pain before or during menstrual bleeding. Respiratory problems. Likes to travel.

Menopause Cell Salts

Kali sulph: lacking self-confidence, moody, hurried, restless.

Nat mur: grief, isolation. Vaginal dryness, especially in menopause. Hair loss. Menopause with genital herpes and/or oral herpes.

Also see Anti-Aging Cell Salts.

About the Author

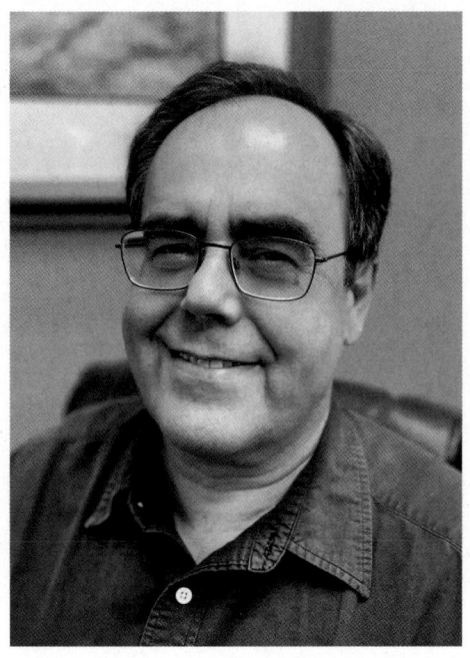

Dave Card has been involved in the health and nutrition industry since 1980. He holds a BA in Psychology, certification as Homeopath, and certification as Master Herbalist. In 1995 Dave started his own business, Dave's Health & Nutrition, which has become a thriving resource in Salt Lake City for all aspects of natural healing and wellness. He consults with clients on a personal basis and has also created unique supplements called Dave's Herbal Formulas. He is a frequent guest speaker at nearby colleges and has published three previous books that have become standards in the field.